Child and
adolescent
services

safeguards for young minds

YOUNG PEOPLE AND PROTECTIVE LEGISLATION

© The Royal College of Psychiatrists 1996

Gaskell is an imprint of the Royal College of Psychiatrists,
17 Belgrave Square, London SW1

British Library Cataloguing-in-Publication Data

A catalogue record for this book is available from the British Library

ISBN 090224194X

SAFEGUARDS FOR YOUNG MINDS

Young People and Protective Legislation

EDITORS

Richard Williams

Richard White

AUTHORS

Richard White

Richard Williams

Anthony Harbour

William Bingley

CONTENTS

CHAPTER 1

THE ORIGINS OF THIS TEXT

1   In 1992, the Royal College of Psychiatrists published the Concise Guide to the Children Act 1989. That slim volume was highly successful and very popular. Consequently, we were asked to edit a second edition. In the course of our deliberations, we have discussed a number of important matters which have a bearing on the management of children and adolescents in mental health services that were not covered in the Concise Guide to the Children Act. Therefore, we decided not just to review, check and update the Concise Guide, but to develop a new text from the original volume. The new title marks the broader scope of this second edition.

2   Readers will find within this volume much that has been drawn from the original Concise Guide. All the text that has been repeated here has been checked and updated and we have added a number of completely new or significantly expanded chapters that respond to the many requests for discussion and advice that we have received from practitioners.

3   It is appropriate to begin by quoting from the foreword to the Concise Guide: *"This volume summarises the major change in the law in England and Wales which took place when the Children Act 1989 received Royal Assent.... One of the consequences of the Act has been to bring together much of the law relating to children, in England and Wales, in a single statute. This is a substantial achievement. The position of children in law has been enhanced and a range of new orders drawn up. The Royal College of Psychiatrists perceived that the changes were such that they would require all professional staff who work with children and families to familiarise themselves with the new concepts and the detailed changes will clearly have a significant impact on the work of a great many psychiatrists."*

THE NEW TEXT

4   This book is concerned with aspects of the law as it applies to the welfare and protection of minors. In particular, it considers the implications for practitioners of:

- the Children Act 1989;

- the Mental Health Act 1983;

- the Mental Health (Patients in the Community) Act 1995;

- the Education Act 1993 and its Code of Practice on Special Educational Needs (1994).

5   The Mental Health Act 1983 has no lower limit of age for most of its provisions and therefore applies to minors as well as adults. In this text, we consider particular issues relating to the use of this legislation with younger people. We do not offer a full account of this Act but make references to its provisions. Readers are referred to Together We Stand (1995) and The Substance of Young Needs (1996) from the NHS Health Advisory Service for a summary of other important legislation.

6   The majority of this book offers a concise summary of the provisions of the Children Act laid out to make relevant information accessible to busy practitioners. We recognise that the law has moved on since 1992, so we have expanded the original text in relevant chapters to highlight

these changes and the developments that have been wrought by case law made in Courts of Record.

THE CONTENTS

7   The original Concise Guide consisted of 11 chapters. We have amalgamated some of them and then added six chapters. Chapter six focuses on matters relating to consent to treatment. Primarily, it draws upon the Children Act 1989 and the Mental Health Act 1983. It explores the issues that affect consent by returning to the legislation itself and subsequent judgements made in Courts of Record. Also, that chapter deals with matters that are of recurrent concern to practitioners including, for example, a section on consent to a service for people who misuse substances.

8   Chapter 10 concerns the restriction of liberty and deals with these issues more substantially than did the original concise guide. We recognise that practitioners find this subject confusing and provocative of anxiety and concern.

9   We also recognise the tensions that arise for individual practitioners who try to work within and apply the law appropriately. In particular, we note the uncertainty expressed by legal, healthcare and child care colleagues as to when to use procedures provided by the Children Act 1989 in preference to those provided by the Mental Health Act 1983, and vice versa. To clarify these and other issues, the second half of chapter 10 offers an interpretation rather than simple reiteration of the law. In advising on the occasions and circumstances when clinical practitioners should adopt the provisions of which Act, we set out a series of factors that might be applied to test each circumstance with a view to aiding the best way forward.

10   Chapter 11 includes a commentary on the Mental Health (Patients in the Community) Act 1995, chapter 12 summarises the complaints procedures that arise from the several pieces of legislation, and chapter nine recognises the impact of the Education Act 1993 on the apprehension of special educational need and the rights of children and their parents in this respect.

11   We are grateful to two lawyers – Anthony Harbour and William Bingley – for collaborating to produce this account. Their advice in certain key areas is not intended to be prescriptive. Rather it is offered to inform, to stimulate discussion and to establish some general principles.

12   As an interpretation of the current legal position, we hope that this new volume will prove as helpful as its predecessor, not only to psychiatrists but also to a wide range of child care practitioners and teachers as well as healthcare and local authority managers.

LEGAL ADVICE

13   It is extremely important that all agencies, their managers and individual professionals involved in managing the mental health of children and young people should have ready access to good legal advice. Any general advice in this text cannot replace that. Experience has shown that the opportunity for practitioners and managers to develop relationships with legal practitioners that allow complex legal matters to be explored over time and in relationship to various cases, will benefit not only the

practitioners themselves but also the children and young people in their care. We strongly support the view that consistently available legal advice of this kind is invaluable.

ACKNOWLEDGEMENTS

14   In introducing this new volume, we acknowledge the enormous help and assistance that we have had from colleagues. One of the editors, Richard White, has undertaken most of the detailed work involved in reviewing the original document and then drafting new chapters. Also, we pay tribute to the advice and enduring support of two colleagues, Dr Greg Richardson and Dr Martyn Gay, with whom we have had the pleasure of working closely; and to Anthony Harbour and William Bingley, who have provided specialist legal advice.

15   The original Concise Guide to the Children Act drew upon the work of a number of others who either provided material directly or provided questions from their own experience that we set out to try to answer. We acknowledge, again, the contributions of Ann Gath, Jean Harris Hendriks, David Jones and Caroline Lindsey and, similarly, we renew our recognition of Mr Arran Poyser and of Dr Donald Brooksbank.

Richard Williams
Richard White

January 1996

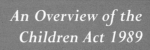

CHAPTER 2

*An Overview of the
Children Act 1989*

INTRODUCTION

16   The Children Act 1989, implemented on 14 October 1991, introduced comprehensive changes to legislation in England and Wales affecting the welfare of children. The Act seeks to reinforce the autonomy of the family through the exercise of parental responsibility; provides for support from local authorities, in particular for families whose children are in need; and legislates for the protection of children who may be suffering or are likely to suffer significant harm. Annual reports on the progress of the Act are published by the Children Act Advisory Committee.

The Aims of the Act

17   The main aims of the Act are:

- to bring together private and public law in one framework;

- to achieve a better balance between the protection of children and the need to enable parents to be able to challenge state intervention;

- to encourage greater partnership between statutory authorities and parents;

- to promote the use of voluntary arrangements;

- to restructure the framework of the courts to facilitate the management of family proceedings.

The Principles of the Act

18   The main principles and provisions embodied in this legislation are that:

- the welfare of children must be the paramount consideration when the courts are making decisions about them;

- the concept of parental responsibility replaces that of parental rights;

- children have increased ability to be parties, separate from their parents, in legal proceedings;

- local authorities are charged with duties to identify children in need and to safeguard and promote their welfare;

- certain duties and powers are conferred upon local authorities to provide services for children and families;

- a checklist of factors must be considered by the courts before reaching decisions;

- orders under this Act should not be made unless it can be shown that this is better for the child than not making an order;

- delay in deciding questions concerning children is likely to prejudice their welfare.

The Scope and Contents of the Act

19   The scope of the Act is extremely wide. Consequently, it is having far-reaching effects and major implications for the practice of all who work with or for children. It changes their standing in law, introduces new

concepts relating to the responsibilities of adults, changes the structure and functioning of the courts, and provides an entirely new range of orders relating to the care of children in both private and public law.

20   The Act is arranged in 12 Parts and 15 Schedules. Particular attention is drawn to Part I which establishes its central concepts.

Part I   *Introductory*
                 This establishes the principle of law that the welfare of children is of paramount importance and the concept of *parental responsibility.*

Part II   *Orders with Respect of Children in Family Proceedings*
                 This establishes a range of orders known as *section 8 orders.*

Part III   *Local Authority Support for Children and Families*
(and   This lays upon the local authority a range of duties and
Schedule 2) powers for the provision of services for children and their families. In particular, it details the law in relationship to the provision of accommodation for children by local authorities and establishes the concept of children being *looked after* by the local authorities.

Part IV   *Care and Supervision*
                 This deals with the provisions concerning care and supervision orders and establishes the *threshold criteria* (see paragraph 42) which must be satisfied before a court can make one of these orders.

Part V   *Protection of Children*
                 This provides for the child assessment order and the emergency protection order.

Part VI   *Community Homes*

Part VII   *Voluntary Homes and Voluntary Organisations*

Part VIII   *Registered Children's Homes*

Part IX   *Private Arrangements for Fostering Children*

Part X   *Childminding and Day Care for Young Children*

Part XI   *The Secretary of State's Supervisory Functions and Responsibilities*

Part XII   *Miscellaneous and General*

KEY CONCEPTS IN THE CHILDREN ACT 1989

Parental Responsibility

21   A central change introduced by the Children Act 1989 was the substitution of the concept of parental responsibility for that of parental rights. The Act defines parental responsibility as *"all the rights, duties, powers, responsibilities and authority which by law the parent of a child has in relation to the child and his property"*. Parental responsibility is given to both the child's father and mother where they are married to each other at, or after, the child's conception. In the case of unmarried parents, the mother has parental responsibility and the father does not have parental responsibility for his child unless he acquires it. This is achieved either by

application of the father to a court or the making of a *parental responsibility agreement* between the father and mother. A guardian who is appointed by the court or by a parent also acquires parental responsibility on taking up appointment (s5).

22   More than one person may have parental responsibility for the same child at the same time, and the person who has parental responsibility will not cease to have that duty solely because some other person subsequently acquires parental responsibility. Parental responsibility is something which parents have and, short of adoption (or freeing for adoption), do not lose.

The Welfare of the Child

23   When a court determines a question with respect to the upbringing of a child, his welfare shall be the court's paramount consideration. Two additional points concerning the welfare of such a child need to be considered.

24   First, the courts are required, in public and private law proceedings, to establish a timetable and give directions for the expeditious handling of each case, because the courts must have regard to the general principle that any delay is likely to prejudice the welfare of the child: s1(2). This is not intended to be rigid. Purposeful delay, as opposed to unplanned drift, is acceptable (C v Solihull Metropolitan Borough Council [1993] 1 FLR 290).

25   Second, courts must have regard, in opposed applications for a section 8 order and in care proceedings, to a check-list concerning the child's circumstances that is set out in s1(3):

- the ascertainable wishes and feelings of the child (considered in the light of his age and understanding);

- his physical, emotional and educational needs;

- the likely effect on him of any change in his circumstances;

- his age, sex, background and any characteristics of his which the court considers relevant;

- any harm which he has suffered or is at risk of suffering;

- how capable each of his parents, and any other person in relation to whom the court considers the question to be relevant, is of meeting his needs;

- the range of powers available to the court in the proceedings in question.

26   This list is known as the *welfare checklist*.

Partnership and Co-operation

27   The major changes in law relating to children that resulted from this Act have their most significant effect upon parents; on others having responsibilities for children; and on local authorities (see The Challenge of Partnership in Child Protection: Practice Guide, HMSO, 1995). Nonetheless, the Act has substantial implications for the NHS and for all healthcare workers who come into contact with children.

28   One of the main themes of this Act is the encouragement of greater co-operation between those responsible for children and statutory or voluntary agencies. Section 27 enables local authorities to request the help of any other authority or person, including health authorities, in relationship to specified actions. Those so requested must comply if the request is compatible with their own statutory duties and obligations and does not unduly prejudice the discharge of any of their functions. At least 18 sections of the Act have implications for health authorities, trusts and for health services staff generally.

29   In the 1980s, the Government published Working Together: A Guide to Arrangements for Inter-agency Co-operation for the Protection of Children from Abuse. A revised, updated edition was published in October 1991 (Home Office, Department of Health, Department of Education and Science & Welsh Office, 1991). See also Child Protection: Medical Responsibilities, Department of Health, HMSO, 1995, an addendum to Working Together.

LOCAL AUTHORITY SERVICES

30   Part III of the Act gives powers and duties to local authorities to provide services for children and their families. Services for children in need and disabled children are brought under one statute. Local authorities are required to produce children's services plans setting out their provision of services under Part III. Health authorities and trusts should be consulted in this process.

Children in Need

31   There is a general duty placed on local authorities to safeguard and promote the welfare of children in their area who are in need and, so far as is consistent with that duty, to promote the upbringing of such children by their families by providing a range and level of services appropriate to those children's needs: s17(1). A child is in need if he is unlikely to achieve or maintain, or to have the opportunity of achieving or maintaining, a reasonable standard of health or development without the provision of services by a local authority under Part III. Equally, he is in need if his health or development is likely to be significantly impaired or further impaired without the provision of such services, or if he is disabled: s17(11).

Children in Local Authority Accommodation

32   Local authorities have a duty to provide accommodation for certain children in need: s20(1). An authority may not provide accommodation if any person with parental responsibility for the child, who is willing and able to provide or arrange accommodation, objects to the authority providing it. Unless another person has a residence order, any person who has parental responsibility may remove the child at any time: s20(7). Local authorities should make agreements with parents or other persons with parental responsibility about the service to be provided in writing, if possible before the service is provided (See the Arrangements for Placement of Children (General) Regulations 1991).

33 Each local authority has duties to the children it looks after (i.e. children accommodated or in care) under ss23 and 24. These include:

- to safeguard and promote his welfare and to make such services available for children cared for by their own parents as appears to the authority reasonable in the case of a particular child;

- to ascertain, as far as practicable, the wishes and feelings of the child, his parents, any other person who has parental responsibility and any other person the authority considers to be relevant, before making any decision with respect to a child they look after or propose to look after;

- to give due consideration, having regard to his age and understanding, to such wishes and feelings of the child as they have been able to ascertain and to his religious persuasion, racial origin and cultural and linguistic background; also to consider the wishes and feelings of any person as mentioned above;

- to advise, assist and befriend him with a view to promoting his welfare when he ceases to be in the local authority's care;

- to provide advice and assistance to qualifying persons between 16 and 21 years old.

34 Where an authority is looking after a child, it must, by s23(2), provide him with accommodation while he is in care, and must:

- maintain him in a children's home (Children's Homes Regulations 1991);

- maintain him in the care of his family, relative or other suitable person (Foster Placement (Children) Regulations 1991);

- maintain him in the care of a parent or person who has parental responsibility (Accommodation of Children with Parents Regulations 1991);

- make other appropriate arrangements which comply with such regulations.

35 As far as is reasonably practicable and consistent with the child's welfare (s23(7) and (8)):

- accommodation should be near the child's home;

- accommodation for a disabled child should not be unsuitable to his needs;

- siblings should be accommodated together.

The Duty of Local Authorities in Respect of Rehabilitation

36 An authority must make arrangements to enable a child to live with his family unless not practical or consistent with his welfare. If he is in care, he may only be placed with parents, or a person with parental responsibility, under strictly controlled conditions: s23.

Case Reviews and Complaints Procedures

37 Under s26, the local authority is required to review the case of each child it looks after, at regular intervals, in accordance with the Review of Children's Cases Regulations 1991.

38   Where a child is being looked after by a local authority, accommodated on behalf of a voluntary organisation or otherwise accommodated in a registered children's home, he will be entitled to use the complaints procedure, also required by s26 and established in accordance with the Representations Procedure (Children) Regulations 1991. Under s26, local authorities must establish and publicise their procedures for considering any representations, including complaints, made by the following:

- a child whom they are looking after or who is not being looked after but is in need;

- a person who qualifies for advice and assistance under s24 (having been looked after);

- a parent or other person with parental responsibility;

- any foster parent;

- such other person whom the authority or voluntary organisation considers has a sufficient interest in the child's welfare to warrant representations being considered by them about the discharge by the authority or voluntary organisation of any of their functions under Part III in relation to the child.

39   The procedure must ensure that at least one person, who is not a member or officer of the authority, takes part in the consideration of the complaint and in any discussions held by the authority about the action to be taken in relation to the child, in the light of the complaint. The authority must have due regard to the findings of those considering the representation and must notify: the child; the person making the representation; and other affected persons of the reasons for its decision and of any action taken or to be taken. While the decision about the child remains with the authority, it may be subject to judicial review if the authority ignores findings or fails to give any satisfactory reasons for its decision.

AN OVERVIEW OF THE ORDERS IN THE CHILDREN ACT 1989

	Children Act 1989	**Previous legislation**
Private Law Orders	Section 8 orders: residence, contact, specific issue, and prohibited steps orders.	Custody, care and control, and access orders.
Public Law Orders	Care, supervision, and education supervision orders.	Care and supervision orders.
	Secure accommodation.	Secure accommodation.
Orders for the Protection of Children	Child assessment, emergency protection, and police protection.	Place of safety order.
Wardship	No longer to be used by local authorities as a route into care, but orders under the inherent jurisdiction of the High Court with or without wardship may be available under s100, except that a child may not be both a ward of court and in care.	Often used to gain the direction of the court when an application for a care order had failed, was not appropriate, or the result was uncertain.

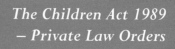

CHAPTER 3

The Children Act 1989
– Private Law Orders

INTRODUCTION

40 Part II of the Act made major changes in the orders available in family proceedings in which questions arise concerning the welfare of children. The concepts of custody, care and control, and access, which had previously caused confusion and misunderstanding, were swept away to be replaced by a range of new provisions. The most important of the private law orders are known as section 8 orders. These are the residence order, contact order, specific issue order and prohibited steps order. Section 8 orders can be made in care proceedings, whether or not the threshold criteria are satisfied, but they cannot be in force at the same time as a care order.

SECTION 8: RESIDENCE ORDER

1   **Definition**

- An order settling the arrangements to be made as to the person with whom a child is to live.

2   **Qualifying Criteria**

- A section 8 order can be applied for separately or as part of other proceedings.

- The court is empowered to make a residence order in any family proceedings.

- No court can make an order that is to have effect beyond the child's 16th birthday unless it is satisfied that the circumstances of the case are exceptional, in which case it may continue until the child becomes 18: s9(6).

- An order can be made even if the child is in local authority care (s9(1)), but the care order is then discharged: s91(1).

3   **Powers and Duties Under the Order**

- A residence order automatically gives the person in whose favour it is made parental responsibility for the child: s12(2).

- When a residence order is in force, no person may either change the child's surname or remove him from the United Kingdom without the written consent of every person who has parental responsibility for the child, or without leave of the court: s13(1).

- A person in whose favour there is a residence order may remove the child for any period less than one month: s13(2).

- The court can make an order:

  - containing directions as to how it is to be put into effect;

  - imposing conditions that must be complied with by any person in whose favour the order is made, who is a parent or has parental responsibility, or with whom the child is living and to whom the conditions are expressed to apply;

  - to have effect for a specified period, or containing provisions which are to have effect for a specified period; or

  - with *"such incidental, supplemental or consequential provision as the court thinks fit"*: s11(7).

4   **Application of General Principles**

- The child's welfare is the court's paramount consideration: s1(1).

- Delay is likely to prejudice the welfare of the child: s1(2).

- There is a presumption of no order unless the court considers that to make an order would be better for the child: s1(5).

- The welfare checklist applies (if the application is opposed); see chapter 3, paragraph 24: s1(4).

5   Who Can Apply?

- There are two categories of applicant: those who can apply as of right and those who require the leave of the court.

As of Right

Any parent including: the unmarried father; a guardian; any person who has a residence order; any party to a marriage, if the child is a child of the family; any person with whom the child has been living for at least three years; a person who has the consent of each person who has a residence order; the local authority, if the child is in care; or, in any other case, each person who has parental responsibility: s10(5).

With Leave

Anyone else, including the child. In the case of a local authority foster-parent, then, unless he is a relative of the child or the child has been living with him for three years within the last five years preceding the application, he must have the consent of the local authority to apply for the court's leave: s9(3).

- For criteria for granting leave, see s10(8) and (9).

- The court is able to make a section 8 order on its own motion, that is, without an application being made: s10(1)(b).

- A local authority may not apply for a residence order: s9(2).

6   Respondents/Notice

- As provided in the Family Proceedings Rules 1991 and the Family Proceedings Courts (Children Act 1989) Rules 1991.

7   Venue

- Magistrates' court, county court or High Court, though this may be limited by a legal aid certificate.

8   Duration

- A residence order ceases to have effect:

    - if the parents live together for a continuous period exceeding six months: s11(5);

    - when the child reaches the age of 16 or, in exceptional circumstances, 18: s91(10).

9   Appeal

- To the High Court from the magistrates' court, and to the Court of Appeal from the county court or High Court.

10   Variation and Discharge

- Any person entitled to apply for a residence order can apply for its variation or discharge. Anyone else shall be entitled to do so if the order was made on his application: s10(6).

- The order is discharged by a care order: s91(2).

SECTION 8: CONTACT ORDER

1   **Definition**

- An order requiring the person with whom a child lives, or is to live, to allow the child to visit or stay with the person named in the order, or for that person and the child otherwise to have contact with each other.

2   **Qualifying Criteria**

- A section 8 order can be applied for separately or as part of other proceedings.

- The court is empowered to make a contact order in any family proceedings.

- No court can make a contact order which is to have effect beyond the child's 16th birthday unless it is satisfied that the circumstances of the case are exceptional: s9(6).

- A section 8 contact order cannot be made in relation to a child in local authority care: s9(1).

3   **Powers and Duties Under the Order**

- The court can make an order:

    - containing directions as to how it is to be put into effect;

    - imposing conditions that must be complied with by any person in whose favour the order is made, who is a parent or has parental responsibility, or with whom the child is living and to whom the conditions are expressed to apply;

    - to have effect for a specified period, or containing provisions which are to have effect for a specified period; or

    - with *"such incidental, supplemental or consequential provision as the court thinks fit"*: s11(7).

4   **Application of General Principles**

- The child's welfare is the court's paramount consideration: s1(1).

- Delay is likely to prejudice the welfare of the child: s1(2).

- There is a presumption of no order unless the court considers that to make an order would be better for the child: s1(5).

- The welfare checklist applies (if the application opposed): s1(4).

5   **Who Can Apply?**

- As with a residence order, there are two categories of applicant: as of right and with leave of the court.

    As of Right

- Any parent including: the unmarried father; a guardian; any person who has a residence order; any party to a marriage, if the child is a child of the family; any person with whom the child has been living for at least three years; a person who has the consent of each person who has a residence order; the local authority, if the child is in care; or, in any other case, each person who has parental responsibility: s10(5).

With Leave

Anyone else including the child. In the case of a local authority foster-parent, then, unless he is a relative of the child, or the child has been living with him for three years preceding the application, he must have the consent of the local authority to apply for the court's leave: s9(3).

- For criteria for granting leave, see s10(8) and (9).

- In addition, the court is able to make a section 8 order on its own motion, that is, without an application being made: s10(1) (b).

- A local authority may not apply for a contact order under this section: s9(2).

6 Respondents/Notice

- As provided in the Family Proceedings Rules 1991 and the Family Proceedings Courts (Children Act 1989) Rules 1991.

7 Venue

- Magistrates' court, county court or High Court, though this may be limited by a legal aid certificate.

8 Duration

- A contact order ceases to have effect:

  - if the parents live together for a continuous period exceeding six months: s11(6);

  - when the child reaches the age of 16 or, in exceptional circumstances, 18: s91(10).

9 Appeal

- To the High Court from the magistrates' court, and to the Court of Appeal from the county court or High Court.

10 Variation and Discharge

- Any person entitled to apply for a contact order can apply for its variation or discharge. Anyone else shall be entitled to do so if the order was made on his application or if he is named in the contact order: s10(6).

- The order is discharged by a care order: s91(2).

SECTION 8: SPECIFIC ISSUE ORDER

1   **Definition**

- An order giving directions for the purpose of determining a specific question which has arisen, or which may arise, in connection with any aspect of parental responsibility for a child, for example medical treatment, education, religion.

2   **Qualifying Criteria**

- A section 8 order can be applied for separately or as part of other proceedings.

- Subject to the following restrictions, the court is empowered to make a specific issue order in any family proceedings:

  - no court can make an order that is to have effect after the child is 16, or, in exceptional circumstances, 18: s9(6);

  - a specific issue order cannot be made in relation to a child in local authority care: s9(1);

  - the court cannot make a specific issue order with a view to achieving a result that could be achieved by a residence or contact order, or in any way that is denied to the High Court by s100(2): s9(5).

3   **Powers and Duties Under the Order**

- The court can make an order:

  - containing directions as to how it is to be put into effect;

  - imposing conditions that must be complied with by any person in whose favour the order is made, who is a parent or has parental responsibility, or with whom the child is living and to whom the conditions are expressed to apply;

  - to have effect for a specified period, or containing provisions which are to have effect for a specified period; or

  - with such *"incidental, supplemental or consequential provision as the court thinks fit"*: s11(7).

4   **Application of General Principles**

- The child's welfare is the court's paramount consideration: s1(1).

- Delay is likely to prejudice the welfare of the child: s1(2).

- There is a presumption of no order unless the court considers that to make an order would be better for the child: s1(5).

- The welfare checklist applies (if the application is opposed): s1(4).

5   **Who Can Apply?**

- There are two categories of applicant:

As of Right

Any parent or guardian. Any person who has a residence order in relation to the child: s10(4).

With Leave

Anyone else, including the child.

- For the criteria for granting leave, see s10(8) and (9).

- The court is able to make a section 8 order on its own motion, that is, without an application being made: s10(1)(b).

6   Respondents/Notice

- As provided in the Family Proceedings Rules 1991 and the Family Proceedings Courts (Children Act 1989) Rules 1991.

7   Venue

- Magistrates' court, county court or High Court, though this may be limited by a legal aid certificate.

8   Duration

- Until a further order is made or until the child is 16 or, in exceptional circumstances, 18.

9   Appeal

- To the High Court from the magistrates' court, and to the Court of Appeal from the county court or High Court.

10   Variation and Discharge

- Any person entitled to apply for a specific issue order can apply for its variation or discharge.

- Anyone else shall be entitled to do so if the order was made on his application: s10(6).

- The order is discharged by a care order: s91(2).

SECTION 8: PROHIBITED STEPS ORDER

1　**Definition**

- An order that no step, that could be taken by a parent in meeting his parental responsibility for a child, of a kind specified in the order, shall be taken by any person without the consent of the court. Orders of this kind might be used to restrain a person with parental responsibility from taking a child out of the country, raising the child in a specified religious denomination, or agreeing to certain specified forms of medical assessment or treatment.

2　**Qualifying Criteria**

- A section 8 order can be applied for separately or as part of other proceedings.

- The court is empowered to make a prohibited steps order in any family proceedings.

- No court can make an order that is to have effect after the child is 16 or, in exceptional circumstances, 18: s9(6).

- A prohibited steps order cannot be made relating to a child in local authority care: s9(1).

- The court cannot make a prohibited steps order with a view to achieving a result that could be achieved by a residence or contact order, or in any way that is denied to the High Court by s100(2): s9(5).

3　**Powers and Duties Under the Order**

- The court can make an order:

　- containing directions as to how it is to be put into effect;

　- imposing conditions that must be complied with by any person in whose favour the order is made, who is a parent or has parental responsibility, or with whom the child is living and to whom the conditions are expressed to apply;

　- to have effect for a specified period, or containing provisions which are to have effect for a specified period; or

　- with such *"incidental, supplemental or consequential provision as the court thinks fit"*: s11(7).

4　**Application of General Principles**

- The child's welfare is the court's paramount consideration: s1(1).

- Delay is likely to prejudice the welfare of the child: s1(2).

- There is a presumption of no order unless the court considers that to make an order would be better for the child: s1(5).

- The welfare checklist applies (if the application is opposed): s1(4).

5　**Who Can Apply?**

- There are two categories of applicant:

As of Right

Any parent or guardian. Any person who has a residence order in relation to the child: s10(4);

With Leave

Anyone else including the child. However, the court will not grant an order on the application of a local authority where it considers it should be making an application for a care or supervision order (Nottinghamshire County Council v P [1993] 2 FLR 134).

- For the criteria for granting leave, see s10(8) and (9).

- The court is able to make a section 8 order on its own motion, that is, without an application being made: s10(1)(b).

6   Respondents/Notice

- As provided in the Family Proceedings Rules 1991 and the Family Proceedings Courts (Children Act 1989) Rules 1991.

7   Venue

- Magistrates' court, county court or High Court, though this may be limited by a legal aid certificate.

8   Duration

- Until a further order is made or until the child is 16 or, in exceptional circumstances, 18.

9   Appeal

- To the High Court from the magistrates' court, and to the Court of Appeal from the county court or High Court.

10   Variation and Discharge

- Any person entitled to apply for a prohibited steps order can apply for its variation or discharge.

- Anyone else shall be entitled to do so if the order was made on his application: s10(6).

- The order is discharged by a care order: s91(2).

SECTION 16: FAMILY ASSISTANCE ORDER

1　**Definition**

An order providing for a probation or local authority officer to advise, assist and befriend a person named in the order.

2　**Qualifying Criteria**

- The court may only make a family assistance order if:

  - it has the power to make an order under Part II (note, that it does not have to make a Section 8 order); and

  - the circumstances of the case are exceptional; and

  - it has obtained the consent of every person named in the order other than the child: s16(3)

3　**Powers and Duties Under the Order**

- The order requires either a probation officer or an officer of the local authority to be available to advise, assist and (where appropriate) befriend any person named in the order: s16(1).

- The persons who can be named in the order are:

  - any parent or the guardian of the child;

  - any person with whom the child is living or in whose favour a contact order is in force with respect to the child;

  - the child.

- Any person named in the order can be required to take such steps as may be specified to keep the officer informed of the address of any person named and to allow the officer to visit such a person(s).

- The order was intended to provide for short-term supervision without the requirement of proving the criteria under s31. It seems to be of limited value and has had little use.

4　**Application of General Principles**

- The child's welfare is the court's paramount consideration: s1(1).

- Delay is likely to prejudice the welfare of the child: s1(2).

- There is a presumption of no order unless the court considers that to make an order would be better for the child: s1(5).

- The welfare checklist does not apply: s1(4).

5　**Who Can Apply?**

- Only the court on its own motion can make the order.

6　**Respondents/Notice**

- Not applicable.

7　**Venue**

- Magistrates' court, county court or High Court.

8   **Duration**

- The order lasts a maximum of six months, although a new order can be made at the end of this period.

9   **Appeal**

- To the High Court from the magistrates' court and to the Court of Appeal from the county court or High Court.

10   **Variation and Discharge**

- The officer may refer to the court the question of whether a section 8 order should be varied or discharged during the period of a family assistance order: s16(6).

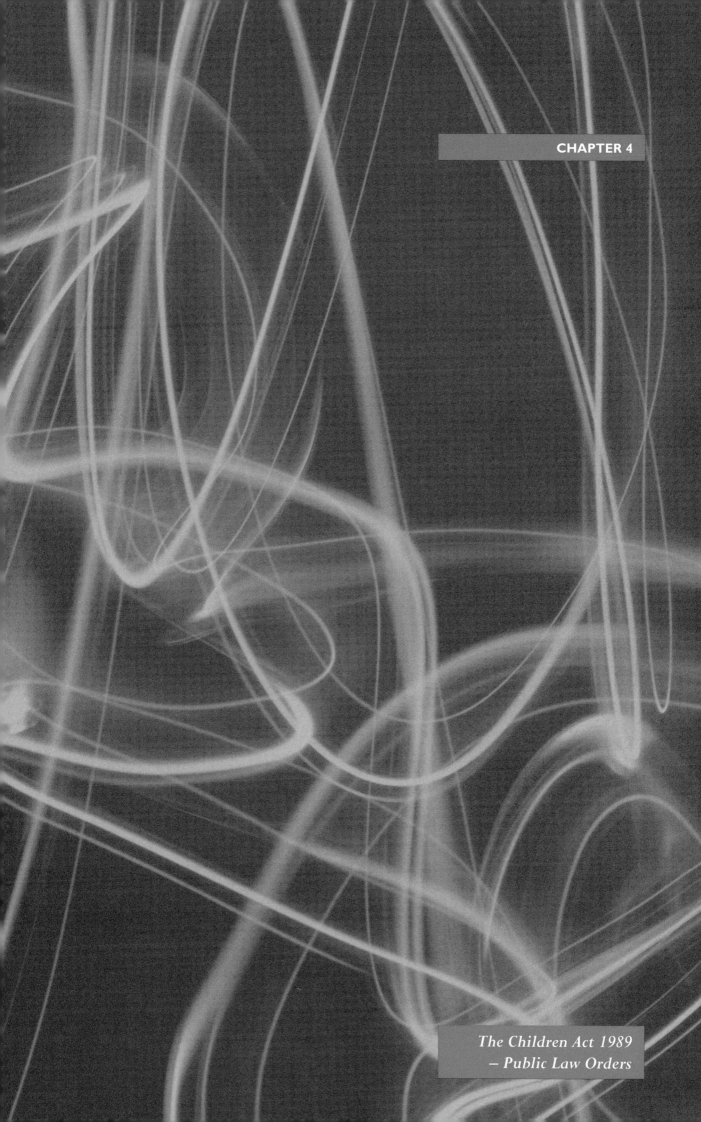

CHAPTER 4

*The Children Act 1989
– Public Law Orders*

INTRODUCTION

41 Part IV establishes the conditions that are required to be satisfied before the court can consider making a care or supervision order.

The Threshold Criteria

42 The courts may only make such orders when satisfied that a child's circumstances meet certain *threshold criteria*. Establishing these criteria involves assessment of the child, his parents' abilities and his circumstances. The criteria and the assessment required are summarised in Figure 1 (page 35) and in a series of steps:

Step 1 Is the child suffering, or likely to suffer, harm by way of ill-treatment, impairment of health or impairment of development?

Step 2 If the harm suffered by a child is that of an effect on the child's health or development, then how does this child's health or development compare with that which could be reasonably expected of a similar child?

Step 3 Is this harm significant?

Step 4 Is this harm or its likelihood attributable to the care given to the child or likely to be given to him if the order were not made?

Step 5 Is the care given to the child not what it would be reasonable to expect a parent to give to him?

Plus

Step 6 Would making an order be better for the child than making no order: s1(5)? Consider the welfare checklist: s1(3). Remember that the welfare of the child is paramount: s1(1).

43 The court has to consider the question of whether a child is suffering significant harm at the time when the local authority acts to protect the child: Re M(A Minor) (Care Order: Significant Harm) [1994] 3 ALL ER 298. Whether harm is likely is a matter for the court. It is not necessary to prove, for example, that harm is more likely to occur than not, but the court does have to be satisfied of the factual basis of the case on a balance of probabilities: Re: H (Threshold Criteria) (Standard of Proof) [1996] 1 FLR 80. The court must also be satisfied that the evidence is cogent and commensurate with the seriousness of the allegations.

Section 1(5)

44 Even if the threshold criteria are satisfied, there remains a further step for courts to consider, that of showing that there are likely to be advantages to the child by making a care or supervision order, which would not accrue if no such order was made. Healthcare practitioners may find themselves called upon, by virtue of their experience, training and clinical activities, to provide written or oral evidence, or to express expert opinion on these issues.

Other Changes to Previous Legislation

45 Care orders are not available for children who fail to attend school (unless they are suffering significant harm) or those facing criminal proceedings before the juvenile courts. The education supervision order is available for those who fail to attend school and, as conditions of supervision orders, the courts may order medical and psychiatric examination and treatment, subject to the consent of the child, where he is deemed capable of understanding.

Figure 1

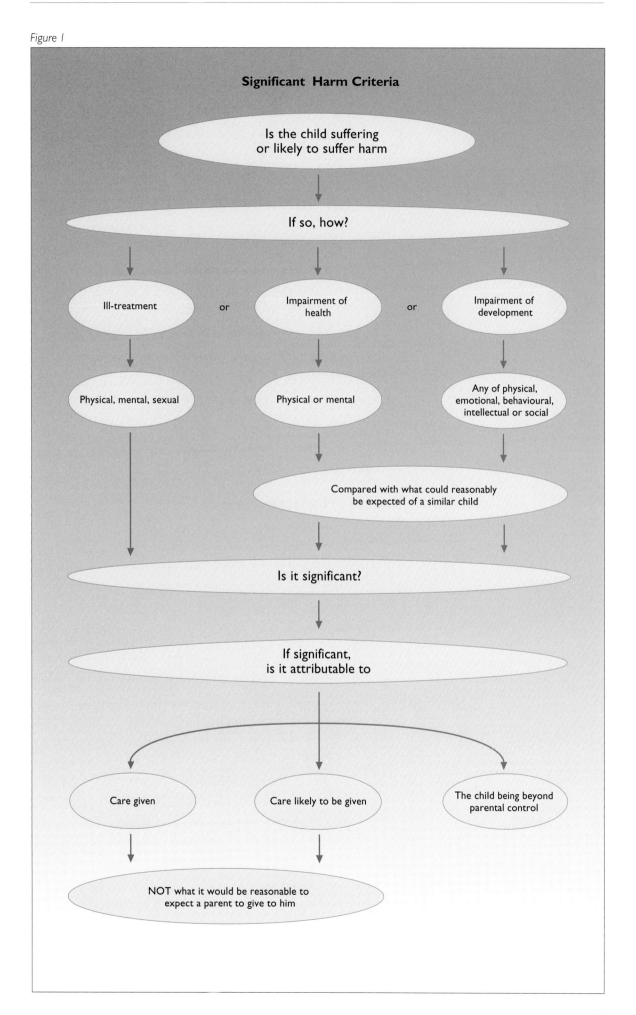

SECTION 31: CARE ORDER

1   **Definition**

A court order giving parental responsibility for a child to a local authority.

2   **Qualifying Criteria**

- The court may only make a care order if it is satisfied:

  - that the child concerned is suffering, or is likely to suffer, significant harm; and

  - that the harm, or likelihood of harm, is attributable to:

    - the care given to the child, or likely to be given to him if the order was not made, not being what it would be reasonable to expect a parent to give him; or

    - the child being beyond parental control: s31(2).

- For elaboration of these criteria see paragraphs 42 to 45 and Figure 1 on page 35.

- Before making a care order, the court must consider the arrangements that the local authority has made, or proposes to make, for affording contact with the child. The court must invite the people involved to the proceedings to comment on these arrangements: s34(11).

3   **Powers and Duties Under the Order**

- The local authority is under a duty to receive the child into its care and to keep him in care while the order remains in force: s33(1). This includes providing accommodation for and maintaining the child: s23(1).

- The local authority acquires parental responsibility for the child (s33(3)(a)), which it shares with the parents: s2(7). However, it can determine the extent to which a parent or guardian of the child may meet their parental responsibility in order to safeguard the child's welfare: ss33(3)(b) and (4).

- There is a presumption of reasonable contact between child and:

  - a parent;

  - a guardian;

  - any person who held a residence order in respect of the child immediately prior to the making of the order;

  - any person who had care of the child under the inherent jurisdiction before the care order was made: ss34(1) and 31(11).

- For specific duties, see ss23 and 24. For specific restrictions on the powers of the local authority under a care order, see s33(5)-(9).

4   **Application of General Principles**

- The child's welfare is the court's paramount consideration: s1(1).

- Delay is likely to prejudice the welfare of the child: s1(2).

- There is a presumption of no order unless the court considers that to make an order would be better for the child: s1(5).

- The welfare checklist applies: s1(3).

In practice, these provisions mean that the local authority will be required to file a care plan at court setting out its proposals for the future care of the child.

5   Who Can Apply?

- A local authority or an *"authorised person"* (the NSPCC): s31(1) and (9).

6   Venue

- To be commenced in the magistrates' court, unless the application arises out of an investigation directed by a higher court or there are relevant existing proceedings in a higher court, but they may be transferred to the county court or High Court: Children (Allocation of Proceedings) Order 1991.

7   Respondents/Notice

- As provided in the Family Proceedings Courts (Children Act 1989) Rules 1991 and the Family Proceedings Rules 1991.

8   Duration

- A care order lasts until the child's 18th birthday unless it is brought to an end earlier: s91(12).

9   Appeal

- To the High Court from the magistrates' court, and to the Court of Appeal from the county court and the High Court.

10   Variation and Discharge

- A care order is discharged by:

  - making a residence order: s91(1);

  - making a supervision order: schedule 3 para 10;

  - the successful application of the child, the local authority or any person with parental responsibility for the child. On such an application, the court can substitute a supervision order for the care order: s39(4).

- A care order is terminated by an adoption order or a freeing order: Adoption Act 1976, ss12 and 18.

SECTION 38: INTERIM CARE ORDER

1   **Definition**

A court order giving parental responsibility for a child to a local authority pending a final hearing.

2   **Qualifying Criteria**

- The court can make an interim care order when adjourning an application for a care or supervision order or giving directions to investigate a child's circumstances under s37(1): s38(1).

- The court may only make an interim care order if it is satisfied that there are reasonable grounds for believing that the circumstances with respect to the child are as mentioned in s31(2): s38(2).

3   **Powers and Duties Under the Order**

- The local authority is under a duty to receive the child into its care and to keep him in care while the order remains in force: s33(1). This includes providing accommodation for and maintaining the child: s23(1).

- The local authority acquires parental responsibility for the child (s33(3)(a)), which it shares with the parents: s2(7). However, it can determine the extent to which a parent or guardian of the child may meet their parental responsibility in order to safeguard the child's welfare: ss33(3)(b)

- There is a presumption of reasonable contact between child and:

  - a parent;

  - a guardian;

  - any person who held a residence order in respect of the child immediately prior to the making of the order;

  - any person who had care of the child by virtue of an order of the High Court under its inherent jurisdiction before the care order was made: ss34(1) and 31(11).

- For specific duties, see ss23 and 24. For specific restrictions on local authority powers under a care order, see s33(5)-(9).

- When it makes an interim order, a court has the power to make directions about medical or psychiatric examination or assessment of the child. The mature minor can refuse to submit to such examination: s38(6).

4   **Application of General Principles**

- The child's welfare is the court's paramount consideration: s1(1).

- Delay is likely to prejudice the welfare of the child: s1(2).

- There is a presumption of no order unless the court considers that to make an order would be better for the child: s1(5).

- The welfare checklist applies: s1(3).

5   Who Can Apply?

- A local authority or an *"authorised person"* (the NSPCC): s31(1) and (9).

6   Venue

- To be commenced in the magistrates' court, unless the application arises out of an investigation directed by a higher court or there are relevant existing proceedings in a higher court, but they may be transferred to the county court or High Court: Children (Allocation of Proceedings) Order 1991.

7   Respondents/Notice

- As provided in the Family Proceedings Courts (Children Act 1989) Rules 1991 and the Family Proceedings Rules 1991.

8   Duration

- Initially, an order can be made for eight weeks with further orders of up to four weeks (longer in the case of orders during the first eight weeks, if the first order was for less than four weeks).

- The court, in determining the period for which the order is to be in force, must consider whether any party who was or might have been opposed to the order was in a position to argue his case in full: s38(10).

- There is no limit to the number of orders that can be made (s38(4) and (5)), though the court must have regard to the delay principle (see above) and must establish a timetable for disposal of the proceedings: s32.

9   Appeal

- To the High Court from the magistrates' court, and to the Court of Appeal from the county court and the High Court.

10   Variation and Discharge

- An interim care order may be discharged on the application of any person with parental responsibility, the child or the local authority (s39(1)) or on the making of a residence order: s91(1).

- Application to discharge a direction may be made by the parties to the proceedings and any person named in the direction.

SECTION 34: CONTACT WITH CHILDREN IN CARE

1   **Definition**

An order requiring a local authority to permit a specified person to have contact with a child in its care.

2   **Qualifying Criteria**

- The child must be in care. There is a presumption that the child in care will be allowed reasonable contact with those entitled to apply for contact: s34(1).

- Before making a care order, the court must consider the arrangements that the local authority has made or proposes to make for affording any person contact with the child and invite the parties to comment on those arrangements: s34(11).

- The court can make an order even though no application for such an order has been made: s34(5).

3   **Powers and Duties Under the Order**

- The court can impose such conditions as it considers appropriate: s34(7).

4   **Application of General Principles**

- The child's welfare is the court's paramount consideration: s1(1).

- Delay is likely to prejudice the welfare of the child: s1(2).

- There is a presumption of no order unless the court considers that to make an order would be better for the child: s1(5).

- The welfare checklist applies: s1(3).

5   **Who Can Apply?**

- The following have a right to apply for an order allowing contact:

    - the child or the local authority;

    - the child's parent or guardian;

    - the person in whose favour a residence order existed immediately prior to the making of the care order.

- Any person who, immediately before the making of the care order, had care of the child by virtue of an order of the High Court under its inherent jurisdiction.

- Anyone else can apply for contact with the leave of the court.

6   **Venue**

- To be commenced in the magistrates' court, unless there are relevant proceedings in a higher court, but they may be transferred to the county court or High Court.

7   Respondents/Notice

- As provided in the Family Proceedings Courts (Children Act 1989) Rules 1991 and the Family Proceedings Rules 1991.

8   Duration

- The order lasts until the child reaches the age of 18 or the date specified in the order, unless discharged.

9   Appeal

- From the magistrates' court to the High Court, and to the Court of Appeal from the county court or High Court.

10   Variation and Discharge

- The child, local authority or person named in the order may apply for variation or discharge: s34(9).

- An order may be varied without a court order in accordance with the provisions set out in the Contact with Children Regulations 1991.

11   Refusal of Contact

- The local authority and the child can apply for an order authorising contact to be refused: s34(4).

- Contact with children in care is ultimately a matter for the court. If the judge concludes that the benefits of contact outweigh the disadvantages of disrupting the local authority's long-term plans which are inconsistent with contact, he must refuse the local authority's application to terminate contact: Re E (A Minor) (Care Order: Contact) [1994] 1 FLR 146.

SECTION 31: SUPERVISION ORDER

1   **Definition**

A court order requiring a local authority or probation officer to advise, assist and befriend a child.

2   **Qualifying Criteria**

- The court may only make a supervision order if it is satisfied:
  - that the child concerned is suffering, or is likely to suffer, significant harm; and
  - that the harm, or likelihood of harm, is attributable to:
  - the care given to the child, or likely to be given to him if the order were not made, not being what it would be reasonable to expect a parent to give him; or
  - the child being beyond parental control: s31(2).
- For elaboration of these criteria see paragraphs 42 to 45 (pages 33 and 34) and Figure 1 on page 35.

3   **Powers and Duties Under the Order**

- The supervisor is under a duty to:
  - advise, assist and befriend the supervised child;
  - take such steps as are reasonably necessary to give effect to the order; and
  - where the order is not wholly complied with, or the supervisor considers that the order may no longer be necessary, to consider whether or not to apply to the court for its variation or discharge: s35(1).
- The supervision order may require the child to comply with specified directions given by the supervisor and that the responsible person shall take all reasonable steps to ensure that the child complies with those directions: schedule 3 part 1.
- The court can include a requirement concerning the examination or treatment of a child, but it must be satisfied that, where the child has sufficient understanding to make an informed decision, he consents to this and that satisfactory arrangements have been made for the examination or treatment: schedule 3 para 5(5).

4   **Application of General Principles**

- The child's welfare is the court's paramount consideration: s1(1).
- Delay is likely to prejudice the welfare of the child: s1(2).
- There is a presumption of no order unless the court considers that to make an order would be better for the child: s1(5).
- The welfare checklist applies: s1(3).

5 Who Can Apply?

- A local authority or an *"authorised person"*: s31(1) and (9).

6 Venue

- To be commenced in the magistrates' court, unless the application arises out of an investigation directed by a higher court or there are relevant existing proceedings in a higher court, but they may be transferred to the county court or High Court.

7 Respondents/Notice

- As provided in the Family Proceedings Court (Children Act 1989) Rules 1991 and the Family Proceedings Rules 1991.

8 Duration

- The order lasts for one year with a possible extension of up to three years: schedule 3 para 6(1) and (4).

9 Appeal

- From the magistrates' court to the High Court, and to the Court of Appeal from the county court or High Court.

10 Variation and Discharge

- The order may be discharged by:
  - making a care order: s91(3); or
  - the successful application of the child, any person with parental responsibility, or the supervisor: s39(2).

SECTION 36: EDUCATION SUPERVISION ORDER

1   **Definition**

A court order requiring a local education authority to supervise a child to ensure that the child is properly educated.

2   **Qualifying Criteria**

- The court must be satisfied that the child is of compulsory school age and is not being properly educated: s36(3). A child is properly educated only if he is receiving efficient, full-time education suitable to his age, ability and aptitude or any special educational needs he may have: s36(4).

- An education supervision order cannot be made in respect of a child in local authority care: s36(6).

3   **Powers and Duties Under the Order**

- The supervisor is under a duty to advise, assist and befriend, and give directions to the supervised child and his parents in such a way as will, in the opinion of the supervisor, secure the child's proper education: schedule 3 para 12.

- The child, and the parent (if asked), may be required to keep the supervisor informed of any change in address and to allow the supervisor to visit the child wherever he is living: schedule 3 para 16.

- If directions are not complied with, the supervisor must consider what further steps to take in exercise of his powers under the Act: schedule 3 para 12.

- If the child persistently fails to comply with any direction given under the order, the local education authority must notify the local authority, which must investigate the circumstances of the child: schedule 3 para 19.

- A parent who persistently fails to comply with a direction given under an education supervision order is guilty of an offence: schedule 3 para 18.

4   **Application of General Principles**

- The child's welfare is the court's paramount consideration: s1(1).

- Delay is likely to prejudice the welfare of the child: s1(2).

- There is a presumption of no order unless the court considers that to make an order would be better for the child: s1(5).

- The welfare checklist applies: s1(3).

5   **Who Can Apply?**

- A local education authority: s36.

6   **Venue**

- Proceedings start in the magistrates' court but may be transferred to the county court or High Court.

7   Respondents/Notice

- As provided in the Family Proceedings Courts (Children Act 1989) Rules 1991 and the Family Proceedings Rules 1991.

- The local education authority must consult the appropriate social services committee before making an application: s36(8).

8   Duration

- The order lasts for one year. Extension may be made for up to three years and there can be more than one extension: schedule 3 para 15.

- The order automatically ceases on:

  - making a care order;

  - the child reaching school-leaving age.

9   Appeal

- To the High Court from the magistrates' court, and to the Court of Appeal from the county court and the High Court.

10   Discharge

- The child, parent or local education authority can apply for discharge: schedule 3 para 17.

SECTION 38: INTERIM SUPERVISION ORDER

1   **Definition**

A court order requiring a local authority or probation officer to advise, assist or befriend a child pending a final hearing.

2   **Qualifying Criteria**

- The court can make an interim supervision order when:

  – adjourning an application for a care or a supervision order;

  – giving directions to investigate a child's circumstances under s37(1) and s38(1).

- The court shall make an interim supervision order when it makes a residence order in care proceedings, unless the child's welfare will be satisfactorily safeguarded without one (s38(3)). But the court may only make the order if it is satisfied that there are reasonable grounds for believing that the circumstances with respect to the child are as mentioned in s31(2): s38(2).

3   **Powers and Duties Under the Order**

- When it makes an interim supervision order, the court has the power to make directions about medical or psychiatric examination or assessment of the child. The mature minor can refuse to submit to such examination: s38(6).

- Directions under s3 may also be imposed (see Supervision Order) but not those under paragraphs 4 and 5.

4   **Application of General Principles**

- The child's welfare is the court's paramount consideration: s1(1).

- Delay is likely to prejudice the welfare of the child: s(1(2).

- There is a presumption of no order unless the court considers that to make an order would be better for the child: s1(5).

- The welfare checklist applies: s1(3).

5   **Who Can Apply?**

- A local authority or an *"authorised person"*: s3(1) and (9).

6   **Venue**

- To be commenced in the magistrates' court, unless the application arises out of an investigation directed by a higher court or there are relevant existing proceedings in a higher court, but the process may be transferred to the county court or High Court.

7   **Respondents/Notice**

- As provided in the Family Proceedings Courts (Children Act 1989) Rules 1991 and the Family Proceedings Rules 1991.

8   Duration

- An order can initially be made for eight weeks with further orders of up to four weeks (longer in the case of orders during the first eight weeks, if the first order was for less than four weeks).

- The court, in determining the period for which the order is to be in force, must consider whether any party who was or might have been opposed to the order was in a position to argue his case in full: s38(10).

- There is no limit to the number of orders that can be made (s38(4) and (5)), though the court must have regard to the delay principle (see above) and must establish a timetable for disposal of the proceedings: s32.

9   Appeal

- To the High Court from the magistrates' court, and to the Court of Appeal from the county court and the High Court.

10   Variation and Discharge

- An interim supervision order may be varied or discharged on the application of any person with parental responsibility, the child or the supervisor: s39(2).

- A person who is not entitled to apply for the order to be discharged, but with whom the child is living, can apply for the variation of the order in so far as it imposes a requirement that affects that person: s39(3).

CHAPTER 5

*The Children Act 1989
– Orders for the Protection
of Children*

INTRODUCTION

46 Part V of the Act, which concerns the protection of children, introduced the child assessment order, and replaced the place of safety order with the emergency protection order. The place of safety order was an *ex parte* order (on, or in the interests of, one side only), as the emergency protection order can be, but rights of being heard by a court shortly after a successful application for an emergency protection order are afforded to parents by the Children Act 1989. The police have separate powers to protect children. An overview of research on the child protection process has recently been published: Child Protection: Messages from Research (Department of Health, 1995).

THE DUTY TO INVESTIGATE

47 Section 47 imposes duties to investigate on the local authority. Where a local authority is informed that a child, who lives or is found in its area, is the subject of an emergency protection order or is in police protection; or the authority has reasonable cause to suspect that a child who lives or is found in its area is suffering or likely to suffer significant harm; the authority is required to make sufficient enquiries to enable it to decide whether it should take any action to safeguard or promote the welfare of the child. This includes consideration of the provision of Part III services, proceedings under s31 and proceedings under Part V, as set out below.

SECTION 43: CHILD ASSESSMENT ORDER

1 Definition

A court order providing for an assessment of a child who is suspected to be suffering, or likely to suffer, significant harm. This order has been little used in practice.

2 Qualifying Criteria

- The court may make a child assessment order if it is satisfied that:

  - the applicant has reasonable cause to suspect that the child is suffering, or is likely to suffer, significant harm; and

  - an assessment of the state of the child's health or development, or the way in which he has been treated is required to enable the applicant to determine whether or not the child is suffering or is likely to suffer significant harm; and

  - it is unlikely that such an assessment will be made or be satisfactory in the absence of an order: s43(1)(a)-(e).

- The court may also consider whether the more appropriate order in the circumstances is an emergency protection order and, if so, make one, if the criteria are satisfied: s43(3).

3 Powers and Duties Under the Order

- The order requires any person, who is in a position to produce the child, to:

  - produce him to such person as may be named in the order;

  - comply with such directions relating to the assessment of the child as the court thinks fit to specify in the order: s43(6).

- The child can only be kept away from home in accordance with directions and for a period or periods specified in the order, if it is necessary for the purposes of the assessment: s43(9).

- The order authorises any person carrying out the assessment to do so in accordance with the terms of the order, but the mature minor can refuse to submit to such assessment: s43(7) and (8).

4 Application of General Principles

- The child's welfare is the court's paramount consideration: s1(1).

- Delay is likely to prejudice the welfare of the child: s1(2).

- There is a presumption of no order unless the court considers that to make an order would be better for the child: s1(5).

- The welfare checklist does not apply: s1(4).

5 Who Can Apply?

- A local authority or an *"authorised person"*: s43(1).

6 Venue

- To be commenced in the magistrates' court, unless the application arises out of an investigation directed by a higher court or there are relevant existing proceedings in a higher court, but the process may be transferred to the county court or High Court: Children (Allocation of Proceedings) Order 1991.

7   Respondents/Notice

- The applicant shall take such steps as are reasonably practicable to ensure that notice is given to:

    - the child's parents;

    - any person with parental responsibility for the child who is not a parent;

    - any other person caring for the child;

    - any person in whose favour a contact order is in force or who is allowed contact with the child under s34;

    - the child: s43(11).

8   Duration

- The order lasts for a maximum of seven days from a date specified in the order: s43(5).

- There can be no further application for a child assessment order within six months without the leave of the court: s91(15).

9   Appeal

- To the High Court from the magistrates' court, and to the Court of Appeal from the county court and the High Court.

10   Variation and Discharge

- The applicant and any person referred to in s43(11) (see above) may apply for variation or discharge: Family Proceedings Rules 1991, r4.2(2) and Family Proceedings Courts (Children Act 1989) Rules 1991, r2.

SECTIONS 44 AND 45: EMERGENCY PROTECTION ORDER

1   **Definition**

A court order authorising the detention of a child in safe accommodation.

2   **Qualifying Criteria**

- The court may make an emergency protection order if, but only if, it is satisfied that:

  - where the applicant is *any person*, there is reasonable cause to believe that the child is likely to suffer significant harm if he is not removed to accommodation provided by, or on behalf of, the applicant; or he does not remain in the place in which he is being accommodated: s44(1)(a);

  - where the applicant is a local authority, inquiries are being made with respect to the child under s47(1)(b) which are being frustrated because access is unreasonably refused and the applicant has reasonable cause to believe access is required urgently: s44(1)(b);

  - where the applicant is an *authorised person*, the applicant has reasonable cause to suspect that a child is suffering, or is likely to suffer, significant harm, and the applicant is making inquiries which are being frustrated because access is unreasonably refused and the applicant has reasonable cause to believe access is required urgently: s44(1)(c).

3   **Powers and Duties Under the Order**

- The order requires any person who is in a position to produce the child to do so if required: s44(4)(a). It authorises:

  - removal of the child to accommodation provided by the applicant, where necessary, in order to safeguard the welfare of the child: s44(4)(b) and (5)(a);

  - prevention of the removal of the child from a hospital or other place in which he was being accommodated immediately before the making of the order: s44(4)(b)(ii);

  - the applicant to have parental responsibility for the child: s44(4)(c).

- While the order is in force, the court has the power to give directions with respect to:

  - the contact which is or is not to be allowed between the child and any named person;

  - medical or psychiatric examination or other assessment of the child (s44(6)), although the mature minor can refuse to submit to such examination: as s44(7).

- The court may issue a warrant authorising any constable to assist (using force if necessary) any person attempting to exercise powers under an emergency protection order who has been prevented (or is likely to be prevented) from doing so by being refused entry to premises and/or access to the child: s48(9).

4   Application of General Principles

- The child's welfare is the court's paramount consideration: s1(1).

- Delay is likely to prejudice the welfare of the child: s1(2).

- There is a presumption of no order unless the court considers that to make an order would be better for the child: s1(5).

- The welfare checklist does not apply: s1(4).

5   Who Can Apply?

- *"Any person"*, a local authority, or an *"authorised person"*: s44(1).

6   Venue

- Application is normally made to a single magistrate or to a sitting magistrates' court.

- The county court or High Court, where that court has directed an investigation or is hearing relevant proceedings, has power to make the order.

7   Respondents/Notice

- With the consent of the justices' clerk, the application may be made without notice to a single magistrate.

- The Family Proceedings Court (Children Act 1989) Rules 1991 give detailed requirements with regard to notice (if it is possible in the circumstances) and the giving of information after the order has been made.

8   Duration

- The order lasts a maximum of eight days, with the possibility of an extension for a maximum of a further seven days if *"the court has reasonable cause to believe that the child concerned is likely to suffer significant harm if the order is not extended"*: s45(4)-(6).

- Irrespective of these limits, the child must be returned as soon as it is safe to do so: s44(10).

- Where the eight-day period ends on Christmas Day, Good Friday, a bank holiday, or a Sunday, the court may specify a period ending at noon on the first later day: s45(2).

9   Appeal

- There is no appeal against any matter relating to an emergency protection order: s45(10) (as amended by the Courts and Legal Services Act 1990 schedule 14) and Essex County Council v F [1993] 1 FLR 847.

10 Discharge

- Application to discharge may be made on one day's notice by the child, a parent, or other person having parental responsibility, or any person with whom the child was living immediately before the making of the order: s45(8).

- No application to discharge may be heard within the first 72 hours of the order (s45(9), nor can there be an application for the discharge of an extended emergency protection order: s45(11).

- A person cannot apply for discharge if he was given notice of the original hearing and was present at the hearing: s45(11).

11 Variation

- Application may be made for variation of a direction (s44(9)), by the parties, the guardian *ad litem*, the local authority in whose area the child is ordinarily resident, and any person named in the direction: Family Proceedings Rules 1991, r4.2(4) and Family Proceedings Courts (Children Act 1989) Rules 1991, r2.

SECTION 46: POLICE PROTECTION

1   **The Power**

- A constable has power under s46 to take a child into police protection.

- He must have reasonable cause to believe that the child would otherwise be likely to suffer significant harm.

- He may remove the child to suitable accommodation or take steps to prevent his removal.

2   **Duration**

- The child may not be kept in police protection for more than 72 hours.

- If it is necessary to extend the period, application must be made for an emergency protection order.

SECTION 50: RECOVERY ORDER

1   Definition

A court order directing the production of a child or the disclosure of his or her whereabouts.

2   Qualifying Criteria

- The court may make an order where it has reason to believe that the child:

  - has been unlawfully taken or kept away from the responsible person named in an emergency protection order or care order, or from police protection;

  - has run away or is staying away from the responsible person; or

  - is missing: s50(1).

3   Powers and Duties Under the Order

- The recovery order:

  - operates as a direction to anybody in a position to do so to produce the child on request to any authorised person;

  - authorises the removal of the child by any authorised person;

  - requires any person who has information about the whereabouts of the child to disclose that information if asked to do so by a constable or officer of the court;

  - authorises a constable to enter premises specified in the order and search for the child, using reasonable force if necessary: s50(3).

4   Application of General Principles

- The child's welfare is the court's paramount consideration: s1(1).

- Delay is likely to prejudice the welfare of the child: s1(2).

- There is a presumption of no order unless the court considers that to make an order would be better for the child: s1(5).

- The welfare checklist does not apply: s1(4).

5   Who Can Apply

- A person with parental responsibility by virtue of an emergency protection order or a care order, or, where the child is in police protection, the designated officer: s50(4).

6   Venue

- Proceedings are commenced in the magistrates' court unless the application arises out of a court-directed investigation, but it may be transferred to the county court or High Court.

7   **Respondents/Notice**

- As provided in the Family Proceedings Courts (Children Act 1989) Rules 1991 and the Family Proceedings Rules 1991.

8   **Duration**

- Until enforcement.

9   **Appeal**

- To the High Court from the magistrates' court, and to the Court of Appeal from the county court and the High Court.

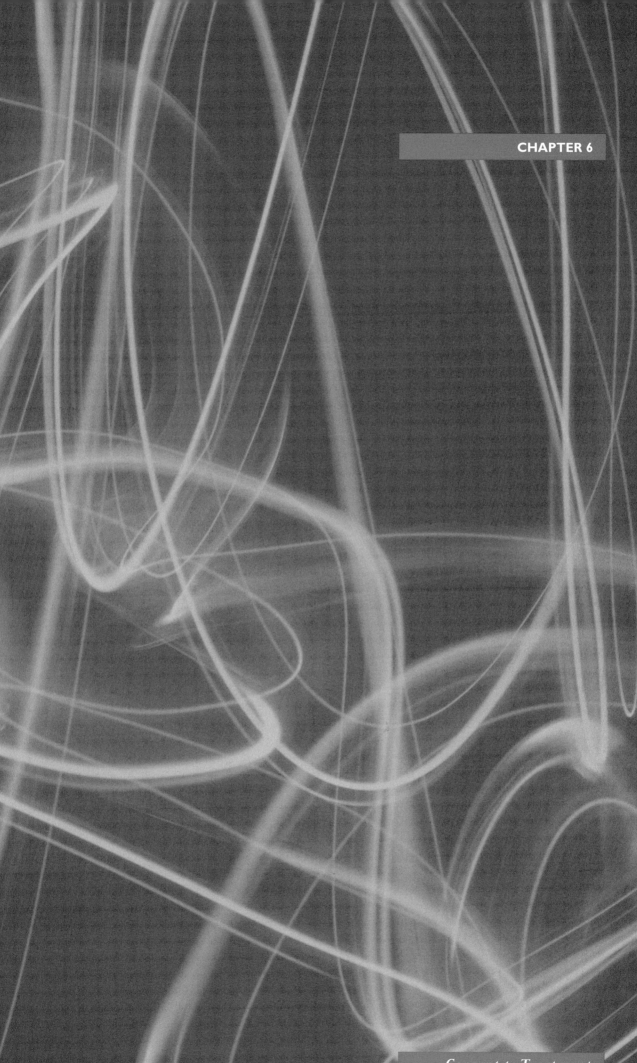

CHAPTER 6

Consent to Treatment

PARENTAL RESPONSIBILITY

48 The Children Act 1989 introduced the concept of *parental responsibility*, emphasising that the duty to care for the child and to raise him to moral, physical and emotional health is the fundamental task of parenthood. Prior to the Act, case law had established that, the older the child, the less extensive parental responsibility may become. Lord Denning observed in Hewer v Bryant, *"the legal right of a parent ends at the 18th birthday, and even up till then, it is a dwindling right which the courts will hesitate to enforce against the wishes of the child, the older he is. It starts with a right of control and ends with little more than advice."*

49 The House of Lords in Gillick v West Norfolk and Wisbech Area Health Authority [1986] AC 112 emphasised that the parental power to control a child exists not for the benefit of the parent but for the benefit of the child. Lord Scarman said: *"Parental rights clearly do exist, and they do not wholly disappear until the age of majority ..... But the common law has never treated such rights as sovereign or beyond review and control. Nor has our law ever treated the child as other than a person with capacities and rights recognised by law. The principle of the law ... is that parental rights are derived from parental duty and exist only so long as they are needed for the protection of the person and property of the child ... parental rights yield to the child's right to make his own decisions when he reaches a sufficient understanding and intelligence to be capable of making up his own mind on the matter requiring decision."*

A CHILD'S CONSENT TO MEDICAL TREATMENT

50 Although, in an emergency, a doctor may undertake treatment if the well-being of the child could suffer by delay, it is normal practice to obtain the consent of a parent as an exercise of their parental responsibility. There may be circumstances, however, in which the child will decide for himself.

The Position of Young People Aged 16 or 17

51 Section 8(1) of the Family Law Reform Act 1969 provides that a child of 16 years or over may consent *"to any surgical, medical or dental treatment which, in the absence of consent, would constitute a trespass to his person, (and the consent) shall be as effective as it would be if he were of full age; and where a minor has by virtue of this section given an effective consent to any treatment it shall not be necessary to obtain any consent for it from his parent or guardian."*

The Position of Children and Young people Aged Under 16

52 In certain circumstances, a child of sufficient age and understanding, who is under the age of 16, can give valid consent. In the Gillick case, it was held that a doctor may lawfully prescribe contraception for a girl under 16 years of age without the consent of her parents. She could have legal capacity to give a valid consent to contraceptive advice and treatment including medical examination. Whether she gave a valid consent in any particular case would depend on the circumstances, including her intellectual capacity to understand advice. There is no absolute parental right requiring the parent's consent to be sought.

53   Speaking of medical treatment generally, Lord Scarman said: *"It will be a question of fact whether a child seeking advice has sufficient understanding of what is involved to give a consent valid in law. Until the child achieves the capacity to consent, the parental right to make the decision continues save only in exceptional circumstances. Emergency, parental neglect, abandonment of the child, or inability to find the parents are examples of exceptional situations justifying the doctor proceeding to treat the child without parental knowledge and consent, but there will arise, no doubt, other exceptional situations in which it will be reasonable for the doctor to proceed without the parent's consent."*

54   Applying this to contraceptive advice and treatment he said, *"There is much that has to be understood by a girl under the age of 16 if she is to have legal capacity to consent to such treatment. It is not enough that she should understand the nature of the advice which is being given: she must also have a sufficient maturity to understand what is involved."*

55   Lord Fraser established five preconditions which would justify a doctor prescribing contraceptive treatment:

- that the girl (although under 16 years of age) will understand his advice;

- that he cannot persuade her to inform her parents or to allow him to inform the parents that she is seeking contraceptive advice;

- that she is very likely to begin or to continue having sexual intercourse with or without contraceptive treatment;

- that unless she receives contraceptive advice or treatment her physical or mental health or both are likely to suffer; or

- that her best interests require him to give her contraceptive advice, treatment or both without the parental consent.

Refusal of Consent

56   Although the Gillick decision might have been taken to imply that a Gillick-competent child could also veto any proposed treatment, Lord Donaldson MR has since said in Re R (A Minor) (Wardship: Medical Treatment) [1992] Fam 11, CA that this is not so. According to his Lordship, all that was decided in the Gillick case was that a competent child could give a valid consent, not that such a child could withhold consent. This approach was followed in Re W (A Minor) (Medical Treatment) [1993] Fam 64, CA, in which it was further held that section 8 of the Family Law Reform Act 1969 does not empower 16 or 17 year-olds to veto medical treatment. In most cases, the consent of somebody with parental authority, be it a parent or local authority, will be sufficient, and application to the court should not be necessary: Re K, W and H (minors) (Consent to Treatment) [1993] 1 FLR 854.

THE POWERS OF LOCAL AUTHORITIES

57   Where a care order is in force, the local authority has parental responsibility and may give consent. The parent retains responsibility and, as a matter of good practice, should still be consulted. If the child is accommodated, the local authority does not automatically have parental responsibility, although the parent may have delegated responsibility to the authority on the child's entry to accommodation. In the absence of

any responsibility, the local authority could seek a court direction under section 8 of the Children Act or through the exercise of the inherent jurisdiction of the High Court.

THE POWERS OF THE COURTS

58 A decision by a parent to consent or refuse to consent to an operation may be overridden by the court: Re C (A Minor) (Medical Treatment) [1993] Fam 64, [1992] 4 All ER 627, CA. It is more likely that the court would find that a child refusing essential treatment would not be Gillick-competent.

59 Where a child has made an informed decision to refuse treatment, but his condition has become life-threatening or seriously injurious, certain statutory provisions, for example where the child is subject to a supervision order, would appear to give the child the right to override a court order for treatment. However, the court may make an appropriate order. In Re J (a Minor) (Medical Treatment) [1992] 2 FLR 165, the Court of Appeal held that treatment of a minor for anorexia could be authorised against her wishes, though the decision about treatment was one for the doctor.

60 In Re C (A Minor) (Wardship: Medical Treatment) [1990] Fam 26, CA, it was held that, where a ward of court was terminally ill, the court would authorise treatment to relieve the ward's suffering.

CONSENT TO MEDICAL OR PSYCHIATRIC EXAMINATION OR ASSESSMENT

61 The Children Act 1989 provides that the court may direct that a child undergo a medical or psychiatric examination or other assessment if one of four orders are in force:

- an emergency protection order, under section 43;

- a child assessment order, under section 44;

- an interim care order, under section 38(6);

- a supervision order, under section 35.

62 The provisions also state that, notwithstanding the court direction, the child who is of sufficient understanding to make an informed decision can refuse to submit to the examination or assessment. It has been held that the High Court, in the exercise of its inherent jurisdiction, can override the child's refusal to consent under section 38(6): South Glamorgan County Council v W and B [1993] 1 FLR 574.

CONSENT TO A SERVICE FOR PEOPLE WHO MISUSE SUBSTANCES

63 Questions on the provision of drugs, or material in conjunction with the use of drugs, such as needles or syringes, could come within the Gillick principles. Careful thought will need to be given in each case as to how the provision and operation of, for example, a needle and syringe exchange can be justified as a medical treatment.

64 The five preconditions which emerge from the Gillick case, could be applied to the provision of a service related to problems of substance misuse:

- that the young person (although under 16 years of age) will understand the advice;

- that the young person cannot be persuaded to inform his or her parents or to allow them to be informed that the young person is seeking drug advice or treatment;

- that the young person is very likely to begin or to continue using drugs with or without the advice or treatment;

- that unless the young person receives advice or treatment on the use of drugs, his or her physical or mental health or both are likely to suffer; and

- that the young person's best interests require the adviser to give advice and/or treatment without parental consent.

65 Valid consent would be ineffective if the prescription of drug advice or treatment were in itself a criminal offence. Therefore, it is important for any adviser to ensure that the actions involved in the treatment are not themselves capable of interpretation as a criminal offence, for example as drug-pushing. If the adviser is to avoid possible prosecution for being an accessory to the unlawful use of drugs, there must be an honest intention to act in the best interests of the young person.

66 The Gillick decision requires that any action should be based on a proper assessment of the circumstances of the case. It refers to assessment by a doctor and clinical judgement, but, when dealing with the mental health of children, a competent assessment may be made by others. An adviser must be able to show the competence to analyse and carry out a reasoned application of the Gillick criteria. It is particularly important to maintain the records to evidence the advice.

THE IMPLICATIONS OF THE MENTAL HEALTH ACT 1983 AND ITS CODE OF PRACTICE

Introduction

67 The Mental Health Act 1983, among other things, regulates the imposition of medical treatment for mental disorder on most detained patients. Part IV of the Act applies to patients admitted for assessment; to the treatment (see paragraph 115 and 116 onwards) of most patients admitted to hospital from the courts under the Act; and to patients transferred from prison under the Act. It sets out requirements and safeguards before certain medical treatments for mental disorder (in particular, electro-convulsive therapy (ECT) and the administration of medication for mental disorder) can be administered in the absence of the patient's valid consent.

68 As there is no age limit to admission under the Act, in certain circumstances children and young people will be detained under its provisions and Part IV will apply.

69 **The Mental Health Act Code of Practice,** *published pursuant to Section 118(4), contains guidance about medical treatment generally (chapter 15) and Part IV of the Act (chapter 16). It also contains a chapter (chapter 30) specifically about children and young people under the age of 18. Currently, the contents of chapter 30 of the* **Code of Practice** *are still official guidance but the authors of this text advise that*

the guidance and information contained in that chapter should be read with extreme caution as it is no longer up-to-date or wholly accurate. It is understood that the Mental Health Act Commission, in pursuit of its responsibilities, will be submitting suggested amendments to the **Code of Practice,** *to Ministers in June 1996 and that these will include a substantial re-draft of chapter 30. Thereafter, it will be for the Secretary of State to consider such amendments for possible inclusion in a revised version of the Code that is planned for publication in 1997. It is suggested that readers may wish to read the present version of chapter 30 of the* **Code of Practice** *in conjunction with this text as this will indicate to them how and in what ways events have overtaken the* **Code of Practice.**

70   The Code of Practice sets out, in paragraph 30.3, principles that should guide practice for this age group:

- young people should be kept as fully informed as possible about their care and treatment; their views and wishes must always be taken into account;

- unless statutes specifically override, young people should generally be regarded as having the right to make their own decisions (and, in particular, treatment decisions) when they have sufficient understanding and intelligence;

- any intervention in the life of a young person considered necessary by reason of their mental disorder should be the least restrictive possible and result in the least possible segregation from family, friends, community and school;

- all children and young people in hospital should receive appropriate education.

71   The Code of Practice continues in paragraph 30.4: *"Whenever the care and treatment of somebody under the age of 16 is being considered, the following questions (amongst many others) need to be asked:*

- *which persons or bodies have parental responsibility for the child (to make decisions for the child)? It is essential that those responsible for the child or young person's care always request copies of any court orders (wardship, care order, residence order [stating with whom the child should live], evidence of appointment as a guardian, contact order, etc) for reference on the hospital ward in relation to examination, assessment or treatment;*

- *if the child is living with either of the parents who are separated, whether there is a residence order and, if so, in whose favour;*

- *what is the capacity of the child to make his own decisions in terms of emotional maturity, intellectual capacity and psychological state?*

- *where a parent refuses consent to treatment, how sound are the reasons and on what grounds are they made?*

- *could the needs of the young person be met in a social services or educational placement? To what extent have these authorities exhausted all possible alternative placements?*

- *how viable would the treatment of an under 16 year-old living at home be if there was no parental consent and no statutory orders?"*

Consent to Medical Treatment of Young People Who Are Admitted or Who Attend Informally

72 The Code of Practice contains guidance (para 30.7) about consent to treatment in the circumstances of young people who are not detained by using powers provided by the Mental Health Act 1983. The advice is out-of-date and inaccurate and is therefore not included.

Parents/Guardians Consent

73 The fact that a child or young person has been informally admitted at the instigation of, or with the consent of his or her parents or guardians should not lead professionals to assume that they have consented to any treatment regarded as necessary. Consent should be sought for each aspect of the child's care and treatment as it arises. Blanket consent forms must not be used (see para 30.8 of the Mental Health Act Code of Practice).

CHAPTER 7

*Hospital Inpatient
Treatment*

INTRODUCTION

74   There are two important provisions in the Children Act 1989 which have consequences for inpatient and day patient mental health units.

- Health authorities and trusts which intend to provide, or do provide, accommodation for a child for a consecutive period of three months or more are required to notify the responsible social services department (sections 85 and 86).

- The Children (Secure Accommodation) Regulations 1991 extend the application of section 25 of the Children Act, which relates to the restriction of children's liberty, to children accommodated by the NHS and who are not detained under the provisions of the Mental Health Act 1983. Even if children are placed in a secure unit by their parents, without any local authority involvement, then the provisions of section 25 will apply.

75   The Mental Health Act 1983 Code of Practice has been amended as a result of these Regulations.

INFORMAL ADMISSION TO HOSPITAL BY PARENTS OR GUARDIANS

76   *The advice in the paragraphs of the* **Code of Practice** *referred to below should be read with great caution, especially when it refers to the limitations on the right of a hospital to admit a competent but objecting child informally (in this context, the* **Code** *means admission other than under the Mental Health Act 1983 or the Children Act 1989) when, in certain circumstances, the consent of the person with parental authority may be sufficient authority.*

77   Paragraphs 30.5 and 30.6 of the Code of Practice to the Mental Health Act 1983 advise as follows:

Children and Young People Aged Under 16

Parents or guardians may arrange for the admission of children under the age of 16 to hospital as informal patients. Where a doctor concludes, however, that a child under the age of 16 has the capacity to make such a decision for himself, there is no right to admit him to hospital informally or to keep him there on an informal basis against his will: (but see Re R (A Minor) (Wardship Consent to Treatment) [1991] 3 W L R 592). Where a child is willing to be admitted, but the parents or guardians object, their views should be accorded serious consideration. It should be remembered that recourse to law to stop such an admission could be sought.

Young People Aged 16 and 17

Anyone in this age group who is *"capable of expressing his own wishes"* can admit or discharge himself as an informal patient to or from hospital, irrespective of the wishes of his parents or guardian: (but see Re W (A Minor) (Medical Treatment: Court's Jurisdiction) [1992] 3 W L R 758).

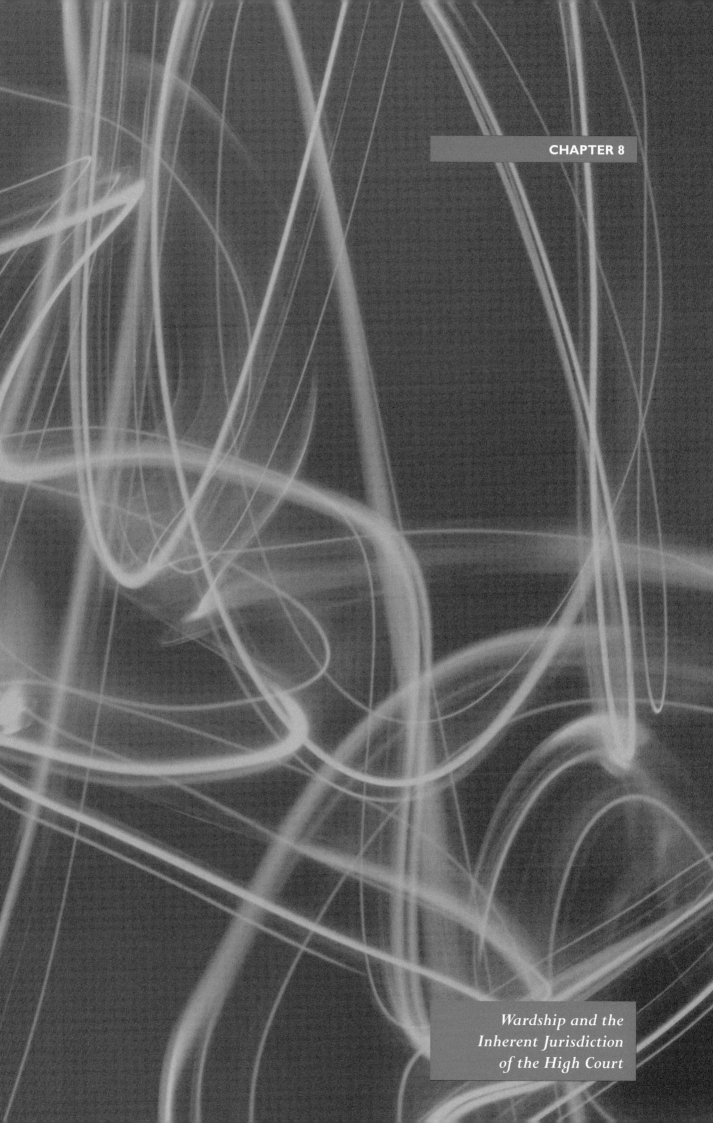

CHAPTER 8

*Wardship and the
Inherent Jurisdiction
of the High Court*

78   The Children Act 1989 has no specific effect on private law wardship, save that the availability of section 8 orders should reduce the need for its use.

79   In the public law field, the changes are considerable. Section 100(1) and (2) provide that there can be no committal to care or supervision under the Family Law Reform Act 1969, s7 or under the inherent jurisdiction of the High Court. Section 31 must be used. The court has no power to require a local authority to accommodate a child and no power to confer on a local authority the power to determine any aspect of parental responsibility: s100(2)(b) and (d). No child, who is the subject of a care order, may be made a ward of court: s100(2)(c). This means that local authorities, working with parents, are responsible for exercising parental responsibility for children in care, and do not seek guidance from or become subject to review by the court in difficult cases.

80   A local authority may, with the consent of the High Court, apply for the exercise of the inherent jurisdiction, if the result it wishes to achieve cannot be achieved by any other means and if there is reason to believe that the child is likely to suffer significant harm if the jurisdiction is not exercised: s100(4) and (5). This might arise in cases which concern an application to override a child's or young person's refusal to consent to medical treatment where no other consent is available (see Re R (A Minor) (Wardship: Medical Treatment) [1992] Fam 11). It might also arise in the instance of injunctions to prevent invasion of a child's privacy, sterilisation, abortion, and any other matters not covered by s8.

81   It is important to note the difference between the immediate effect of wardship, in which the court is responsible for all important decisions concerning the child, and which remains available where the child is not in care, and the exercise of the inherent jurisdiction, which has no effect until there is a court order.

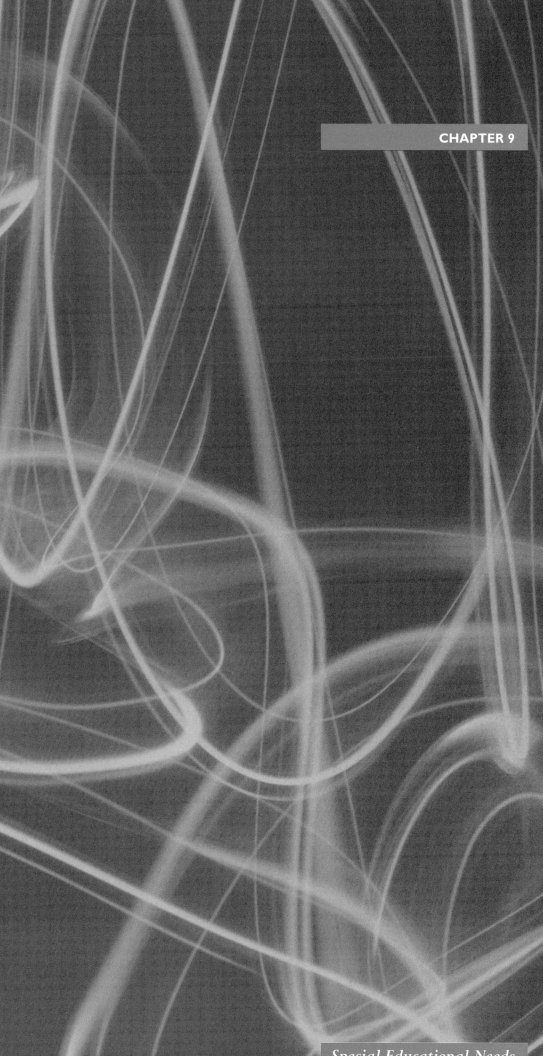

CHAPTER 9

Special Educational Needs

82 Under the Education Act 1993, local education authorities, and funding authorities for grant-maintained schools, must have regard to the need for securing that special provision is made for pupils with special educational needs.

83 A child has special educational needs if he has a learning difficulty. This means he:

   • has significantly greater difficulty in learning than the majority of children of the same age; or

   • has a disability which either prevents or hinders him from making use of educational facilities of a kind provided for children of the same age in schools within the area of the local education authority; or

   • is under five and falls within (a) or (b) or would do so if the special educational provision was not made for the child.

84 The Education Act 1993 contains duties to identify, assess and provide for those with such needs. This may involve a multi-disciplinary assessment in consultation with parents. Mental health professionals may be involved at any stage of the process in advising, assessing or giving evidence.

85 The Education Act 1993 establishes a Code of Practice which sets out detailed guidance. It identifies a continuum of need to be dealt with in five stages, extending from action within the school to the making of a statement of special educational needs requiring a specific provision.

86 Parents have a right of appeal to an independent tribunal under sections 169 to 173 against:

   • a refusal to make an assessment;

   • a decision not to make a statement;

   • the content of a statement;

   • a refusal to reassess a child with a statement.

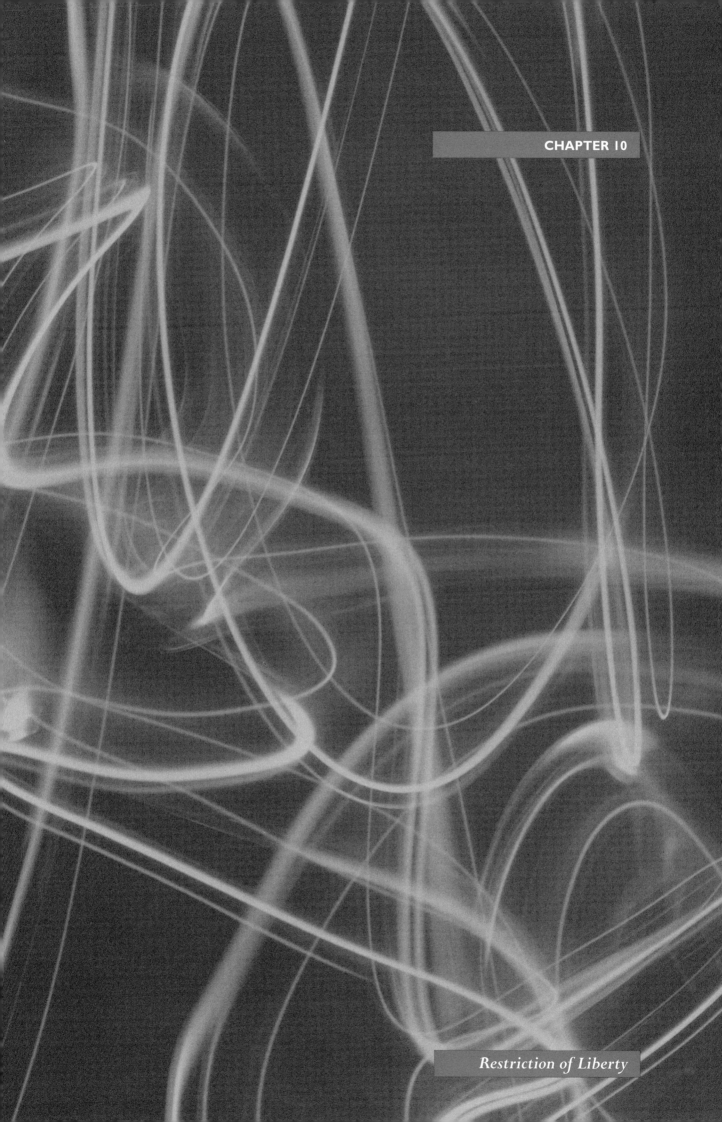

CHAPTER 10

Restriction of Liberty

THE STATUTORY BASIS - THE CHILDREN ACT 1989

87　　The liberty of children may only be restricted in accordance with provisions set out in section 25 of the Children Act 1989, the Children (Secure Accommodation) Regulations 1991, and the Children (Secure Accommodation) No 2 Regulations 1991. The Children Act 1989 Guidance and Regulations, Volume 4, Residential Care (Department of Health 1991, referred to subsequently as the Guidance, Volume 4) supplements the statutory provisions. Secure tracking units are not considered here, since, at the time of writing, the provisions relating to them had not come into force.

88　　Secure accommodation is defined as accommodation provided for the purpose of restricting liberty (section 25(1) of the Children Act 1989). The Guidance recognises that the interpretation of this term is ultimately a matter for the court, but states: *"it is important to recognise that any practice or measure which prevents a child from leaving a room or building of his own free will may be deemed by the court to constitute restriction of liberty. For example, while it is clear that the locking of a child in a room, or part of a building, to prevent him leaving voluntarily is caught by the statutory definition, other practices which place restrictions on freedom of mobility (for example, creating a human barrier), are not so clear cut."* (Guidance, Volume 4, para 8.10).

89　　The use of secure accommodation by local authorities in respect of children looked after by them and for children accommodated by health authorities, NHS trusts and local education authorities and children accommodated in children's homes, nursing homes and mental nursing homes, is permitted only where the criteria in section 25 of the 1989 Act are fulfilled.

90　　Local authorities have a duty under the Children Act 1989 to take reasonable steps to avoid placing children within their area in secure accommodation (Schedule 2, para 7). The guidance states: *"Restricting the liberty of children is a serious step which must be taken only when there is no appropriate alternative. It must be a `last resort' in the sense that all else must first have been comprehensively considered and rejected - never because no other placement was available at the relevant time, because of inadequacies in staffing, because the child is simply being a nuisance or runs away from his accommodation and is not likely to suffer significant harm in doing so, and never as a form of punishment ... Secure placements, once made, should be only for so long as is necessary and unavoidable. Care should be taken to ensure that children are not retained in security simply to complete a pre-determined assessment or 'treatment' programme"* (Volume 4, para 8.5).

91　　Section 25 provides that secure accommodation may not be used in respect of a child unless it appears:

- that he has a history of absconding and is likely to abscond from any other type of accommodation; and

- that if he absconds, he is likely to suffer significant harm; or

- that if he is kept in any other type of accommodation he is likely to injure himself or other persons.

92　　A child may only be kept in secure accommodation for as long as the relevant criteria apply. Furthermore, a child under the age of 13 years shall not be placed in secure accommodation in any children's home without the prior approval of the Secretary of State. Such approval shall be subject to such terms and conditions as the Secretary of State sees fit (reg 4).

93   The maximum period during which a child's liberty may be restricted without the authority of a court is 72 hours, either consecutively or in aggregate in any period of 28 days (reg 10(1) Children (Secure Accommodation) Regulations 1991). There is some relaxation of this restriction to meet difficulties caused by the period expiring on a Saturday, a Sunday or public holiday (reg 10(3) Children (Secure Accommodation) Regulations 1991).

Children to Whom Section 25 of The Act Does Not Apply

94   The restrictions on the use of secure accommodation do not apply to:

- a child detained under any provision of the Mental Health Act 1983 (as these will be provided for by the mental health legislation);

- a child detained under section 53 of the Children and Young Persons Act 1933, concerning the punishment of certain grave crimes.

95   Children accommodated under the following provisions may not have their liberty restricted in any circumstances:

- a young person over 16 who is being accommodated under section 20(5) of the Children Act;

- a child in respect of whom a child assessment order under section 43 of the Children Act has been made and who is kept away from home pursuant to that order.

Applications To Court

96   Applications to court for authority to use secure accommodation may only be made by or on behalf of a local authority looking after a child or, as extended by No.2 regulation, where the child is accommodated by a health authority or NHS trust, by that authority.

97   Application is made to the family proceedings court, except where the matter arises in the context of a case already before a county or High Court, in which case application is made to that court, or to the Youth Court, where criminal proceedings are involved.

98   The criteria applicable to the use of secure accommodation by local authorities is modified in the case of children *looked after* by them who are: a. detained children under the Police and Criminal Evidence Act 1984, s38(6); and b. children remanded to local authority accommodation under the Children and Young Persons Act 1969, s23 but only if:

- the child is charged with, or has been convicted of a violent or sexual offence, or of an offence punishable, in the case of an adult, with imprisonment for a term of 14 years or more; or

- the child has a recent history of absconding while remanded to local authority accommodation, and is charged with, or has been convicted of an imprisonable offence alleged, or found to have been committed while he was so remanded.

99   In these circumstances, secure accommodation may not be used unless it appears that any accommodation other than that provided for the purpose of restricting liberty is inappropriate because:

- the child is likely to abscond from such other accommodation; or

- the child is likely to injure himself or other people if he is kept in other accommodation.

Evidence

100 When considering whether to make an order, the court is under a duty to consider whether the relevant criteria for keeping a child in secure accommodation under section 25 are satisfied. The extent to which the welfare principles under section 1 of the Act have to be taken into account has been a matter for difference of opinion. The Department of Health guidance states: *"It is the role of the court to safeguard the child's welfare from inappropriate or unnecessary use of secure accommodation, both by satisfying itself that those making the application have demonstrated that the statutory criteria in section 25(1) or regulation 6 as appropriate have been met and by having regard to the provisions and principles of s1 of the Act. The court must therefore be satisfied that the order will positively contribute to the child's welfare and must not make an order unless it considers that doing so would be better for the child than making no order at all"* (Guidance, Volume 4, para 5.7).

101 The Court of Appeal has now held that the welfare of the child was relevant but not the paramount consideration and that the principles of section 1 do not apply: Re M (a Minor) (Secure Accommodation Order) [1995] 1 FLR 418, CA. The role of the court was to decide whether the evidence showed that the authority should be given the power to take such a serious step.

102 An order if made, is permissive; it does not require the child to be kept in secure accommodation. Initially, the maximum period of an authorisation is three months. The court should not automatically make an order for three months but must consider what is necessary for the circumstances of the case: Re W (A Minor) (Secure Accommodation Order) [1993] 1 FLR 692. Authorisation may be renewed for further periods of up to six months at a time (regs 11 and 12). An order should be for no longer than is necessary and unavoidable, and may have a short-term usefulness to break a pattern of absconding: W v North Yorkshire County Council [1993] 1 FCR 693.

103 Where an application for a secure accommodation order is made in family proceedings, hearsay evidence is admissible. It is desirable to have a psychiatric report available as evidence: R(J) v Oxfordshire County Council [1992] 3 All ER 660. The court must give reasons for its decision: Family Proceedings Court (Children Act 1989) Rules 1991, rule 21.

Accommodating Children and Young People in Secure Accommodation

104 When a child is accommodated by a local authority or health authority, plans should be made for the discharge of the child, when the authorisation to continue to detain the child expires. There may be occasions when the child cannot immediately be accommodated at home or elsewhere. Although plans should be made sufficiently well in advance to ensure that suitable accommodation is available, it would not

seem to be unlawful to permit the child to continue to live on the same premises.

105 Provided the child was advised that he could leave the premises, if he so wishes, it would appear that he would not come within the provision of being 'kept' within accommodation provided for the purpose of restricting liberty.

106 It is appropriate to re-state a general principle here that if a child is accommodated as described in the previous paragraph in secure provision, then any person who has parental responsibility may remove the child from such accommodation at any time.

THE STATUTORY BASIS - THE MENTAL HEALTH ACT 1983

107 In certain circumstances, the Mental Health Act 1983 provides an alternative statutory basis for the restriction of a child or young person by way of admission to hospital. In general terms, there is no age limit on detentions under the Mental Health Act.

108 The Act provides four main routes into care in psychiatric hospitals or units.

- Informal Admission (Section 131);

- Civil Admission (Compulsory admission following professional decision - Part II of the Act);

- Court to Hospital (Part III of the Act);

- Prison to Hospital (Part III of the Act).

109 For the purposes of this chapter it is only necessary to consider civil admission and the two principal admission sections.

Assessment - Section 2

110 Any person, including a young person, on the application of an approved social worker (ASW) or nearest relative (NR) and supported by two medical recommendations, may be detained in a hospital under section 2 of the Act for up to 28 days on the grounds that the person:

- is suffering from mental disorder of a nature or degree which warrants the detention of the patient in hospital for assessment (or for assessment followed by medical treatment) for at least a limited period; and

- he or she ought to be so detained in the interests of his or her own health or safety or with a view to the protection of other persons.

Treatment - Section 3

111 Any person including a young person, on the application of an ASW or NR, and supported by two medical recommendations, may be detained, initially for six months, renewable for another six months and thereafter for a year at a time, on the grounds that:

- the person is suffering from mental illness, severe mental impairment, psychopathic disorder or mental impairment, and his mental disorder is of a nature or degree which makes it appropriate for him to receive medical treatment in hospital;

- in the case of psychopathic disorder or mental impairment, such treatment is likely to alleviate or prevent a deterioration of his condition; and

- it is necessary for the health or safety of the patient or for the protection of other persons that he should receive such treatment and it cannot be provided unless he or she is detained under the section.

Review and Consent to Treatment

112 Anybody detained under either of the above two sections acquires the right to apply to a Mental Health Review Tribunal and they are subject to the provisions of Part IV of the Mental Health Act 1983.

CHOOSING BETWEEN THE CHILDREN ACT 1989 AND THE MENTAL HEALTH ACT 1983

Introduction

113 During its reviews of forensic and child and adolescent mental health services between 1992 and 1995, the NHS Health Advisory Service was made aware of the anxieties of professionals about identifying the most appropriate legal framework, in circumstances when it was thought necessary to enforce a child or adolescent's residence in a particular place and/or require them to undergo medical treatment.

114 The choice is not always easy. Current official guidance is sparse and unhelpful. It is hoped that the next edition of the Mental Health Act Code of Practice will be more useful. Given the complex relationship between the two pieces of legislation and evolving relevant case law, it is not possible to provide other than general pointers that could usefully be taken into account by professionals when deciding which route to take.

115 In identifying such pointers, a range of considerations has to be taken into account. The Children Act may appear less stigmatising as it does not specifically refer to mental disorder and its use may be seen as reflecting social and family failure rather than a problem located in the mental health of an individual young person. The Children Act 1989, unlike Part IV of the Mental Health Act 1983, does not provide specific powers to enforce medical treatment, or to safeguard the rights of detained patients. These safeguards include the review of detention by Mental Health Act managers and Mental Health Review Tribunals, and the general oversight of the Mental Health Act Commission.

116 Notwithstanding the above, the Mental Health Act 1983 is not specifically orientated towards children and adolescents and their needs and circumstances. Some may argue that, in other regards, its underlying principles and safeguards are not sufficient to adequately protect the interests of children and young persons in every circumstance in which it would be possible to apply the Act. In addition, it would be unrealistic not to recognise, that for some, being detained under the Mental Health Act 1983 may be perceived as being more stigmatising. While it is difficult to identify any formal stigmatising consequences that flow from having been detained under the Act, there is clearly a risk of informal consequences. In considering such possibilities (for example, having difficulty in gaining employment), it is important to clarify whether the risk is a consequence of having received inpatient mental health care or having been detained under the Act: not infrequently it is the former.

117 An additional consideration is the fact that most lasting powers under the Children Act are consequent upon court decisions, while the exercise of the powers under discussion in this text that are afforded by the Mental Health Act 1983 is the consequence of professional judgement (see paragraphs 115 and 116) and does not involve court review.

118 In evaluating the legal framework within which an individual child should be treated, the breadth of the concept of treatment needs to be understood. Treatment for children and young people may encompass both detention in a secure environment and the imposition of what the lay person would more easily recognise as medical treatments, such as those referred to in Part IV of the Mental Health Act 1983. Unlike the Mental Health Act 1983, the Children Act 1989, does not specifically provide for a child's decision about medical treatment to be overridden. As described in Chapter 6, consent will usually depend on the exercise of parental responsibility. If there is a dispute, the court can make a section 8 order specifying the steps to be taken. (See pages 24 & 25.) In the limited circumstances set out in paragraph 62, where the Children Act does provide that the child who has sufficient understanding to make an informed decision may refuse to undergo a medical or psychiatric examination or assessment, the High Court may be able to make an order overriding the refusal under its inherent jurisdiction. Where the court has made a secure accommodation order under section 25 of the Children Act, the order authorises non-consensual detention in a therapeutic environment, but decisions about treatment must still be dealt with by way of the usual consents.

Underlying Principles

119 Set out below are a set of guiding principles and some pointers that may be helpful for professionals to take into account when considering the appropriate legal framework; especially when it is proposed to treat a child or younger person in the absence of their consent. It is hoped that these suggestions will not only help to ensure that many of the major considerations will be addressed by those responsible for identifying the appropriate legal framework, but that they will also contribute to a national debate about the principles and the considerations that should underlie such decisions.

120 When considering the appropriate legal framework the provider of treatment must, in each case:

- have sufficient understanding of the relevant legal provisions;

- have easy access to competent legal advice;

- keep in mind the importance of ensuring that the child's care and treatment is managed with clarity, consistency and within a recognisable framework;

- attempt to select the least stigmatising and restrictive option that is consistent with the care and treatment objectives for that patient.

Pointers

121 Pointers, derived from the pooled experience of the authors, are outlined in the following paragraphs:

- **Discrimination and Stigma**

  In taking these matters into account, it is important that any judgement is carefully thought through and based upon a realistic assessment of the relevant considerations.

- **Parental Involvement**

  The involvement of those persons having parental responsibility is a factor that will have to be considered. The child can be treated with the consent of any person having parental responsibility. If a child is detained under the Mental Health Act 1983, the parent will usually be the nearest relative and must be consulted about admission. Professionals should consider whether this is desirable where abuse by a parent is alleged. Consulting the nearest relative may not be desirable or therapeutically indicated where there is an allegation of abuse. It may be appropriate to obtain a court order for another person to exercise the functions of the nearest relative.

- **Specific Treatment Decisions**

  Any decision to treat a child or young person should, of course, be discussed with them and with the person having parental responsibility for them, if available. The refusal of the child or young person to be medically treated can be overridden by the consent of the person having parental responsibility. If both refuse and treatment is important, a court order may be sought under section 8 (see pages 24 & 25) or the inherent jurisdiction of the High Court. Such an approach may have the benefit of allowing the specific proposed treatment to be addressed and the wishes of the child to be represented.

- **Due Process**

  Detention under the Mental Health Act 1983 provides a legal framework for control which protects the rights of patients more effectively than overriding a patient's choice by way of the admission and treatment of the child or young person on the authority of somebody with parental authority. In these latter circumstances, there is an absence of procedural and legal safeguards.

  It is important to remember that the provisions of Part IV of the Mental Health Act 1983 afford safeguards when a child or young person's refusal of treatment for mental disorder is being overridden. These safeguards apply to the provision of certain forms of treatment, particularly the administration of medication for mental disorder, after three months, and of ECT.

- **Age Specificity**

  The Mental Health Act 1983 is not age-specific. It does not infantilise and so may allow the treatment provided to be focused on the nature of the illness itself.

- **Assessing the Objectives of the Treatment**

  The specific purpose of the intervention in the child's life needs to be evaluated. For instance, is the objective of the detention assessment or treatment? Relevant considerations include the length of time that the child requires treatment and detention, and the seriousness or longevity of the illness. For example, a very seriously ill adolescent may require treatment within the Mental Health Act 1983, whereas a serious, self-harming offender with a psychiatric component to his or her problem may require detention under the Children Act 1989. The balance in evaluating these particular options lies between the need for containment, and the need for medical treatment for mental disorder.

- **Review and Audit**

  The involvement of the child in any legal process is another important factor to be considered. Under the Children Act 1989, a guardian *ad litem* may be appointed by the court and the application itself will be audited and reviewed in a court setting. In addition, the child may also be represented separately by a solicitor.

  Some have expressed concern about detention under the Mental Health Act 1983, in relation to external review. Although admission under the provisions of this Act can only take place according to specific legal criteria, there is no external audit of the admission process. But the continuing need for detention is externally reviewed by the Mental Health Review Tribunal and the provisions of the Act with regard to consent to treatment apply.

  Both secure accommodation orders under the Children Act 1989 and the powers of detention afforded by the Mental Health Act 1983 are time-limited with established renewal, review and complaint procedures.

CONTROL AND RESTRAINT OF CHILDREN AND YOUNG PEOPLE

122 Questions about treatment of children and young people include those with respect to control and restraint, seclusion, destimulation and 'time-out'. There is little statutory or common law basis for regulating these methods of treatment, and it is necessary to look to general principles. Certainly, practitioners should be aware that any method of treatment involving restraint or restriction of liberty could be subject to the provisions in section 25 of the Children Act 1989. In respect of any method of treatment, the question of informed consent will arise.

123 The Children's Homes Regulations 1991 provide for the conduct of homes and for securing the welfare of children in such homes. The regulations provide for the control and discipline of children in homes. Physical control or restraint of a child must of its nature be at least a technical assault. The authority for the assault must arise through the proper restriction of liberty, self-defence or consent. Reference should also be made to Guidance on Permissible Forms of Control in Residential Care (Department of Health, April 1993).

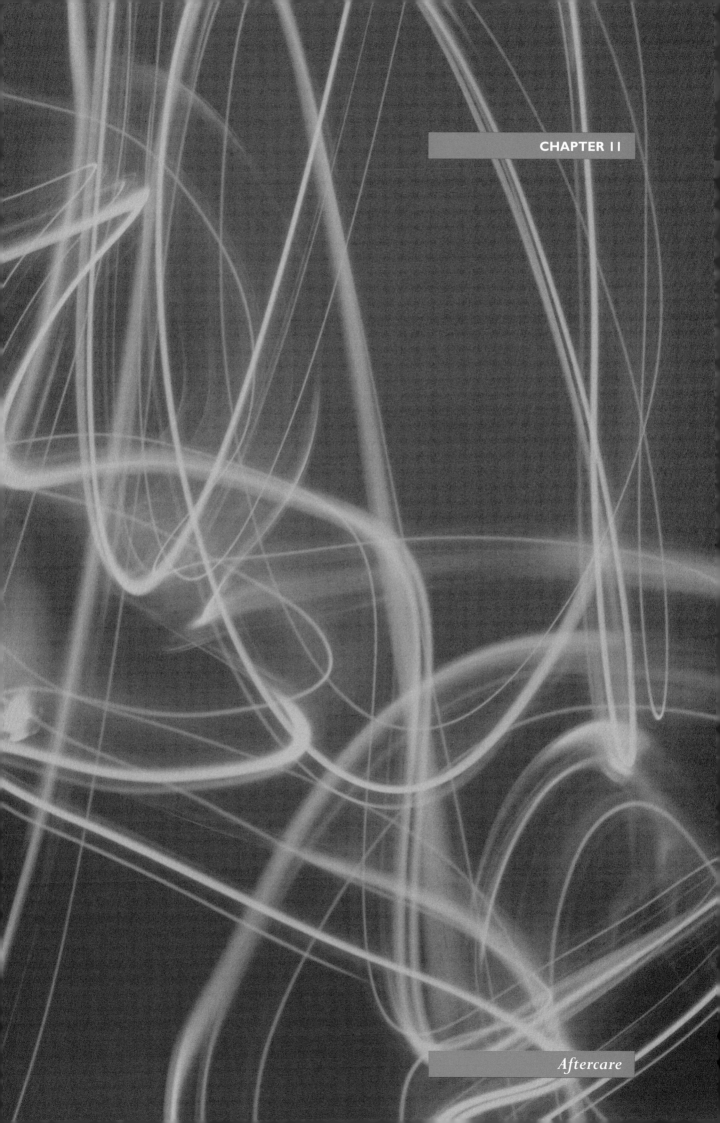

CHAPTER 11

Aftercare

THE CHILDREN ACT 1989

124 Section 24 of the Children Act 1989 provides local authorities with powers and duties to prepare the young people they are looking after for the time when they cease to be so looked after, and to provide aftercare advice and assistance. This applies to any young person under 21 who ceases, after reaching the age of 16, to be looked after by a local authority or accommodated by any health authority, NHS trust or local education authority, or in any residential care home, nursing home or mental nursing home, provided that he was accommodated for at least three months.

125 Before a local authority begins to look after a child, or as soon as practicable afterwards, it shall make immediate and long-term arrangements for placing the child and for promoting the welfare of the child to be placed: the Arrangements for Placement of Children (General) Regulations 1991. Section 23 requires local authorities to provide him with accommodation while he is in their care and to maintain him.

126 These provisions should ensure that a proper admissions policy is in place for every establishment and a plan for every child. The plan should contain the criteria for admission, the objectives of the placement, the way of achieving those objectives, the outcome expectations and the sequel to the placement which should provide a context for aftercare. However, the extent to which these provisions are implemented in practice is questionable.

THE MENTAL HEALTH ACT 1983

127 The Mental Health Act also establishes a duty to provide aftercare for certain categories of detained patients. This duty is imposed jointly on health authorities and social service authorities. The Mental Health Act Code of Practice, para 27.6, refers to the responsibility of the responsible medical officer *"to ensure that a discussion takes place to establish a care plan to organise the management of the patient's continuing health and social care needs"*. Paragraphs 27.7 and 27.8 list who should be involved in the planning process and emphasise the importance of those who are involved being able to take decisions, as far as possible, on behalf of their agencies.

128 Section 117 only establishes a duty in relation to patients who have been detained under the powers afforded by some sections of the Mental Health Act 1983. However, the Care Programme Approach, and the responsibilities of social service departments in relation to care management encompass a larger group of patients who have had contact with the specialist mental health services. This group will include informal patients.

THE MENTAL HEALTH (PATIENTS IN THE COMMUNITY) ACT 1995

129 The Mental Health (Patients in the Community) Act 1995 amended the Mental Health Act 1983, the Code of Practice issued by the Secretary of State and the Mental Health (Scotland) Act 1984. The provisions of this Act became effective on 1 April 1996.

130 The Act:

- makes provision for certain mentally disordered patients in England and Wales to receive aftercare under supervision after leaving hospital, (otherwise called supervised discharge);

- provides for the making of community care orders in the case of certain mentally disordered patients in Scotland;

- amends the law relating to mentally disordered patients absent without leave by extending the period during which they can be returned to hospital;

- amends the provisions relating to leave of absence from hospital for detained patients by enabling it to be granted for up to a year;

- deals with a variety of purposes that are connected with these circumstances.

131 In England and Wales, application for aftercare under supervision may be made by the responsible medical officer (RMO) where a patient:

- is liable to be detained in a hospital in pursuance of an application for admission for treatment;

- and has attained the age of 16 years.

132 The main intention of this Act is that patients should be supervised after leaving hospital, for the period allowed by the Act, with a view to securing that they receive the aftercare services provided for them under section 117 of the Mental Health Act 1983.

133 With respect to Scotland, the Mental Health Act 1995 enables the RMO to make an application to the sheriff for a community care order with respect to a patient who is liable to be detained in a hospital provided that the patient, instead of continuing to be liable to be so detained, be subject to the conditions specified in the order, being conditions imposed with a view to ensuring that he receives:

- medical treatment; and

- aftercare services provided for him under section 8 of the Mental Health (Scotland) Act 1984.

134 The Act details:

- the grounds for applications and the circumstances and conditions that must pertain before each application is granted;

- the requirements on RMOs to consult with other professionals and the patients for whom applications are considered;

- the duties of Health Authorities in England and Wales to consult with the local social services department before they make orders;

- the duties of sheriffs in Scotland with respect to making or refusing orders;

- the duties of the Mental Welfare Commission in Scotland;

- the duration of orders;

- the mechanisms that must be followed for informing patients;

- the procedures for the review and variation of orders and those to be followed when there are changes in key professional appointments;

- the circumstances and conditions in which orders must be renewed or may be ended;

- special provisions as to patients:

    - sentenced to imprisonment;

    - moving from Scotland to England or Wales;

    - moving from England or Wales to Scotland;

    - absent without leave.

135 In each instance, the Act requires:

- in England or Wales, the appointment of;

    - a community responsible medical officer;

    - a supervisor;

- in Scotland, the appointment of:

    - a special medical officer;

    - an aftercare officer.

136 As the Act contains procedures that are to be followed in its application, readers are encouraged to turn to the text of the Act itself, when they consider that the provisions of this Act could be of benefit to patients for whom they have responsibilities.

137 The authors consider that it is likely that very few minors will satisfy the conditions established for aftercare that are found by the Mental Health (Patients in the Community) Act 1995. Relative to adults, few young people are detained in hospital under the provisions of the Mental Health Acts. In England and Wales, there is the further qualification of patients having attained the age of 16 before applications for supervised discharge are lawful.

138 Thus, the provisions of this legislation cannot apply to the great majority of younger people about whom this text has been written. Nevertheless, the Act does apply in full measure to a small number of younger patients who meet the criteria. The editors of this text can envisage its provisions being applied appropriately to enhance the care of certain, carefully selected adolescents. Hence, a review of this recent Act is included. Nonetheless, in the opinion of the editors, this Act throws into greater contrast the relative lack of provision in the mental health legislation for the aftercare of children and adolescents below the age of 16.

139 Passage of time and experience will indicate the applicability and utility of this legislation with adolescents.

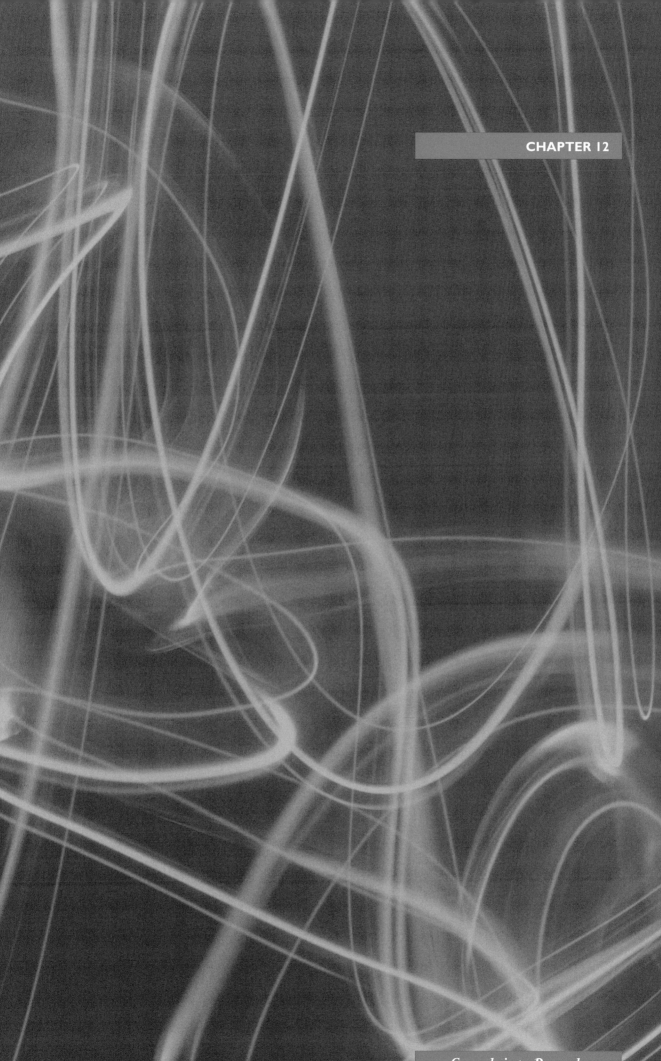

CHAPTER 12

Complaints Procedures

THE CHILDREN ACT 1989

140 Where a child is being looked after by a local authority, accommodated on behalf of a voluntary organisation or otherwise accommodated in a registered children's home, he will be entitled to use the complaints procedure required by section 26 of the Children Act and established in accordance with the Representations Procedure (Children) Regulations 1991.

141 Under section 26 of the Children Act, local authorities must establish and publicise their procedures for considering any representations, including complaints, made by the following:

- a child whom they are looking after, or who is not being looked after but is in need;

- a person who qualifies for advice and assistance under section 24 (having been looked after);

- a parent or other person with parental responsibility;

- any foster parent; or

- such other person as the authority or voluntary organisation consider has a sufficient interest in the child's welfare to warrant representations being considered by them about the discharge by the authority or voluntary organisation of any of their functions under Part III in relation to the child.

142 The procedure must ensure that at least one person who is not a member or officer of the authority takes part in the consideration of the complaint alongside any discussions had by the authority about the action to be taken in relation to the child in the light of the complaint. The authority must have due regard to the findings of those considering the representation and must notify the child, the person making the representation and other affected persons of its reasons for its decision and of any action taken or to be taken. Although the decision about the child remains with the authority, if it ignores findings or fails to give any or any satisfactory reasons, it may be subject to judicial review.

THE HOSPITAL COMPLAINTS ACT 1985

143 Provision is made under the Hospital Complaints Act 1985 for a hospital to establish a complaints procedure.

THE MENTAL HEALTH ACT 1983

144 The Mental Health Act Code of Practice states: *"Children and young people in hospital (both as informal and detained patients) and their parents or guardians should have ready access to existing complaints procedures, which should be drawn to their attention on their admission to hospital. The Managers should appoint an officer whose responsibility it is to ensure that this is done and to assist any complainant."* (para 30.13).

145 The Mental Health Act Commission also has a power to investigate complaints under section 120(1) of the Mental Health Act 1983. This investigative power only exists in relation to detained patients.

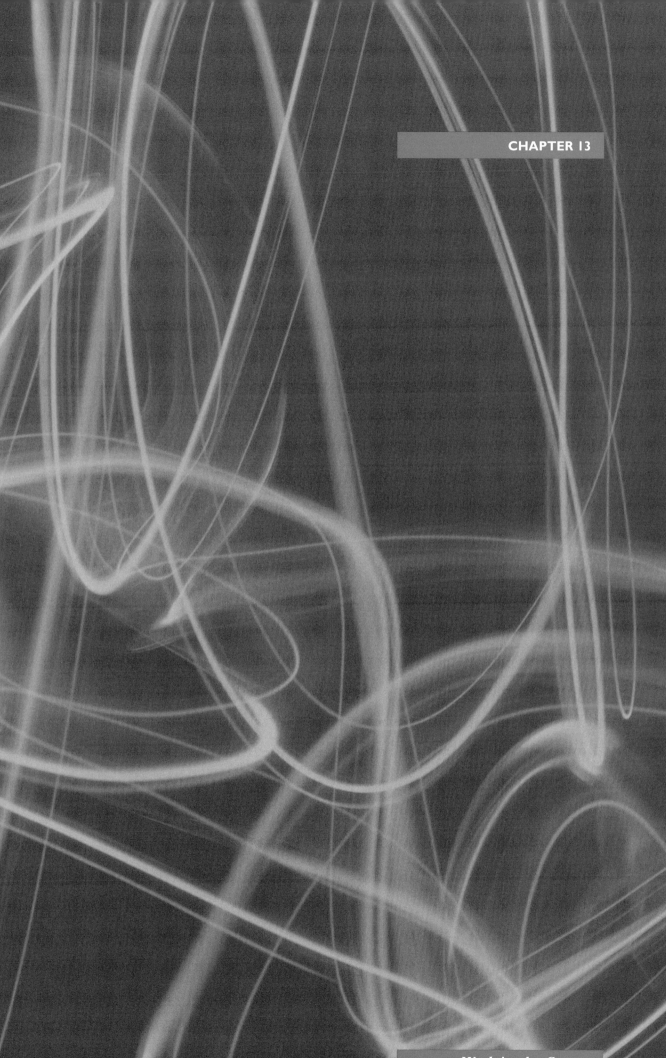

CHAPTER 13

Work in the Courts

INTRODUCTION

146 There are a number of courts that deal with matters relating to children, and in which a child and adolescent psychiatrist and a wide range of other professionals may appear to give evidence of fact, or to give evidence as an expert.

THE COURTS

The Youth Court

147 Following changes made by the Children Act 1989, this court deals solely with juvenile offenders.

The Magistrates' Court

148 Under the Children Act 1989, a family panel of magistrates has powers to deal with family proceedings in the family proceedings courts. The court has a lay bench of two or three magistrates, sitting with a justices' clerk, or a stipendiary magistrate. Magistrates do not have jurisdiction in relation to divorce, wardship and the inherent jurisdiction of the High Court, child abduction and some cases of domestic violence. They do have jurisdiction to make orders concerning children, including orders under Parts II, III and IV of the Children Act 1989 (see above), and those relating to maintenance, adoption and domestic violence between spouses.

The County Court

149 Children Act cases are dealt with at a family hearing centre or a care centre, depending on the nature of the case. Care proceedings allocated from the magistrates' court because of their complexity will be heard at a limited number of nationwide care centres by judges who have had special training for the purpose. The wider range of orders available under the Children Act, and other matters such as residence and contact, divorce and nullity, domestic violence and adoption, can be heard at a family hearing centre.

The High Court

150 Family matters are dealt with in the Family Division either at the Royal Courts of Justice in the Strand in London, or at a district registry. High Court judges or deputies sit alone to hear complex cases under the Children Act 1989. They also hear cases relating to adoption, wardship, the inherent jurisdiction and appeals from the magistrates' court. Certain appeals are to the Divisional Court, when two judges will sit together.

The Court of Appeal

151 Appeals from the High Court and county court go to the Court of Appeal and are heard by two or three Lords Justices of Appeal. There is not always an automatic right of appeal and the leave of the judge may be necessary. Even where there is an automatic right, legal practitioners are warned not to pursue appeals without clear grounds for doing so.

The House of Lords

152 This is the final court of appeal in the United Kingdom and will only hear cases where there is an issue of public importance. Cases are heard before five Law Lords.

153 The High Court, Court of Appeal and the House of Lords are Courts of Record. Each can establish legal precedent, which is binding on courts lower than itself.

EVIDENCE

The Children Act 1989

154 The Children Act 1989 introduced some important changes relating to the evidence of children. The evidence of a child witness in civil proceedings, who does not understand the nature of the oath, can be heard by the court if, in its opinion, the child understands that it is his duty to speak the truth and he has sufficient understanding to justify his evidence being heard: s96(2).

155 The Children (Admissibility of Hearsay Evidence) Order 1993 provides that hearsay evidence shall be admissible in family proceedings in the magistrates' court; also in the county court and the High Court in relation to the upbringing of a child.

156 Section 98 provides that, in care or protection proceedings, no person shall be excused from giving evidence, or answering any question, on the ground that it may incriminate him or his spouse of an offence, and that a statement or admission made shall not be admissible in criminal proceedings other than those for perjury against the person making the statement or his spouse.

Expert Evidence

157 Applications to the court for a secure accommodation order, and under section 31 for a care or supervision order, are likely to require expert evidence. Frequently, this relates to the health or development of the child or a proposed carer, and is particularly relevant to the question as to whether a child is suffering or is likely to suffer significant harm.

158 The mental health expert can find that his expertise is sought from a number of different sources: the local authority; the guardian *ad litem*; or a member of the child's family. If it is the local authority, he may have been involved before legal proceedings are initiated, but may need to continue his involvement afterwards. Otherwise, it is probable that his advice will be sought specifically for the purpose of the proceedings. It is important that clear instructions are obtained as to the purpose of the request for advice; what questions are to be considered; and what the overall context of the case is. (Further guidance on this aspect of the work can be found in Child Psychiatry and the Law, 3rd Edition, Royal College of Psychiatrists, 1996.)

The Roles of Experts

159 The courts have held that experts must only express opinions that they genuinely hold and that are not biased in favour of one party. If an expert does seek to promote a particular case, the report must make that clear,

but that approach should be avoided. A misleading opinion may well inhibit a proper assessment of the case by non-medical professional advisers; it may increase costs and lead parties and, in particular, parents to false views and hopes.

160 A helpful summary of the duties of an expert giving evidence is set out in Re AB (A Minor) (Medical Issues) [1995] 1 FLR 181, extracted as below.

- Expert evidence presented to the court should be (and should be seen to be) the independent product of the expert, uninfluenced as to form or content by the exigencies of litigation.

- An expert witness should provide independent assistance to the court by way of objective, unbiased opinion in relation to matters within his expertise. An expert witness should never assume the role of advocate.

- An expert witness should state the facts or assumptions on which his opinion is based. He should not omit to consider material facts which detract from his concluded opinion.

- An expert witness should make it clear when a particular question falls outside his expertise.

- If an expert's opinion is not properly researched because he considers that insufficient data is available, then this must be stated with an indication that the opinion is no more than a provisional one.

- If after exchange of reports, an expert witness changes his view on a material matter, such change of view should be communicated to the other side without delay and, when appropriate, to the court.

- Where expert evidence refers to photographs, reports or other similar documents, these must be provided to the opposite party at the same time as the exchange of reports.

161 There is increasing pressure on experts to discuss reports with each other prior to the hearing, in an attempt to reach agreement or limit the issues: Re M (Minors) (Care Proceedings: Child's Wishes) [1994] 1 FLR 749. Directions should be given by the court to ensure that sufficient time is set aside for expert evidence: Re MD and TD (Minors) (Time Estimates) [1994] 2 FLR 336. The parties and the court should have an understanding of the issues involved at any directions hearing.

Funding

162 It is also important to establish the basis for funding an expert witness. If expert advice is sought by a local authority, in or out of court, the expert should establish whether work is expected to be done under the National Health Service or by separate payment. If the request for an expert opinion comes from the guardian *ad litem* for the child or a solicitor for a member of the family, it may be that financial arrangements will have to be made, outside any National Health Service provision. Funding may then be provided through the legal aid system.

Disclosure of Confidential Information

163 Any person can be required by *sub poena* or witness summons to produce documents at court, notwithstanding that it may be confidential information about a patient. In order to ensure that this is available before the trial, it may be required by pre-trial order.

164 The House of Lords held, in Re L (a Minor) (Police investigation: Privilege) [1996] Times, March 22, that the privilege attached to reports by third parties and prepared on the instructions of a client for the purposes of litigation could be set aside. This was held to be distinct from legal professional privilege attaching to communications between a solicitor and a client which should be allowed to be absolute. The court has a discretion not to order disclosure, and may decline to do so, especially in the interests of a child.

165 There is some uncertainty over the power of the court to override professional privilege and order disclosure of medical reports, where the identity of the author of the report or the source of the reports is not known. The most favoured view at present is that set out by Mr Justice Thorpe in Essex County Council v R (Legal professional privilege) [1993] 2 FLR 826. He held that legal representatives having reports relevant to the determination of a matter concerning children, but contrary to the interests of their client, had a positive duty to disclose the reports to all the parties and to the courts. This view may now be questioned in the light of Re L.

Witness Credibility

166 The question concerning whether an expert witness can give evidence to a court about whether a child is telling the truth has produced different responses from the Court of Appeal. At the time of going to press, the cumulative effect of recent decisions in Re N (a Minor) (Child Abuse: Evidence) (1996) Times, March 25 and Re M and R (Minors) (Transcript, 21 May 1996) appears to be as follows:

- An expert witness may give evidence about whether a child is telling the truth, but the relevance of that evidence and the weight to be attached to it is a matter for the judge.

- A video recording of the evidence of a child was admitted as a form of hearsay evidence. It was for the judge to decide its weight and credibility. He would judge the internal consistency and inconsistency of the story. He would look for any inherent improbabilities in the truth of what the child related and would decide what part, if any, he could believe.

- The judge would receive expert evidence to explain and interpret the video recording. This would cover such things as the nuances of emotion and behaviour, the gestures and the body movements, the use or non-use of language and its imagery, the vocal inflections and intonations, the pace and pressure of the interview, the child's intellectual and verbal abilities, or lack of them, and any signs or the absence of signs of fantasising.

- It was for the judge to separate admissible from inadmissible expert evidence. Evidence from an expert might best be couched in terms that a particular fact was consistent or inconsistent with sexual abuse, and that it rendered the child's evidence capable or incapable of being accepted by the judge as true.

- Evidence of a diagnosis of sexual abuse called for a very high level of expertise. For the court to rely on opinion evidence, even to admit it, the qualifications of the witness must extend beyond experience gained as a social worker and require clinical experience as or akin to a child psychologist or child psychiatrist.

LEGAL ADVICE

167 It is important that all agencies and individual professionals involved in managing the mental health of children and young people should have ready access to good legal advice. This should include legal advice competent to consider both mental health and children's legislation. In some cases, the mental health expert will only be an adviser or witness to action being taken by another agency. In those circumstances, the advice and guidance of their legal advisers may be sufficient. In other cases, the expert may need to have access to legal advice for the purposes of his own agency or if he is unsure about what he is being asked to do. The availability of that expertise and the different professional perspective is an essential benefit to the provision of an appropriate service. Knowledge and understanding of the legal framework should lead to better informed decision-making on policy and on individual cases. Ultimately, better all-round understanding should enable improvements in the legal system itself to be brought about.

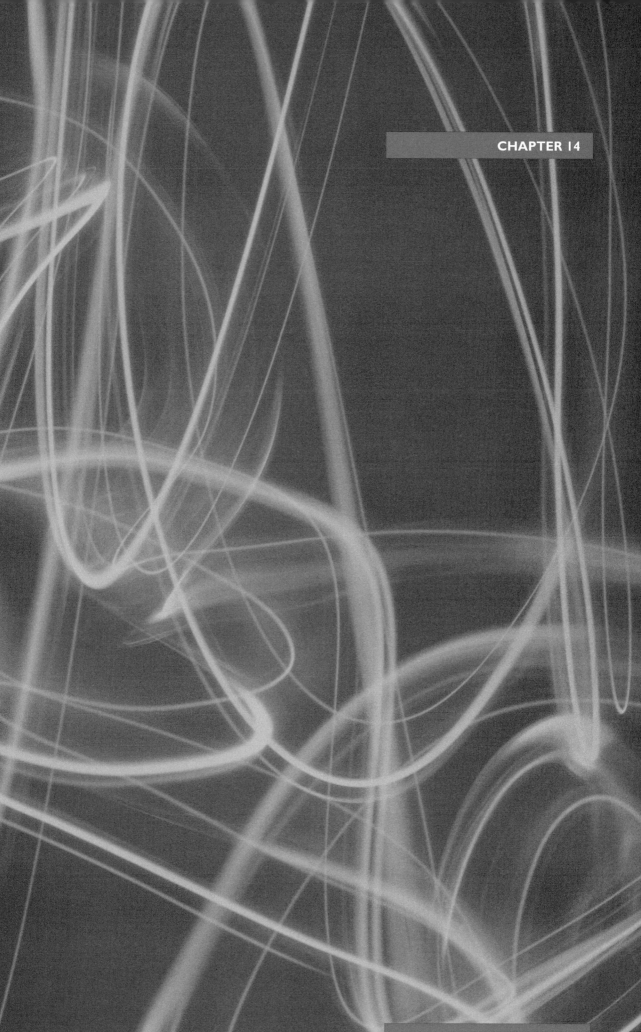

CHAPTER 14

*Further Reading and
Bibliography*

FURTHER READING

168 Despite the growing number of explanatory texts, the Children Act 1989, as amended, along with Regulations and Orders issued by the Secretaries of State in pursuance of their duties, remain the only truly authoritative sources of information on what is or is not lawful in relation to children. Rules of court are contained in a number of orders by the Lord Chancellor's Department (1991a, b, c).

169 A similar situation can be said to exist with respect to the Mental Health Act 1983 and the Mental Health (Patients in the Community) Act 1995. The Code of Practice for the Mental Health Act 1983 has been referred to in various chapters in this text. For the most part, it remains authoritative. Nonetheless, informed sources regard its advice with respect to children and adolescents as out-of-date and not wholly accurate (see pages 66, 67 and 71). It is understood that Chapter 30 of the Code of Practice, which relates to children and adolescents is being re-drafted. Therefore, readers are advised to consider with great caution the advice in the Code of Practice with respect to children and adolescents.

170 In 1991, HMSO published detailed Guidance and Regulations on the Children Act 1989 in nine volumes:

Volume 1   *Court Orders*

Volume 2   *Family Support, Day Care and Education Provision for Young Children*

Volume 3   *Family Placements*

Volume 4   *Residential Care*

Volume 5   *Independent Schools*

Volume 6   *Children with Disabilities*

Volume 7   *Guardians Ad Litem and Court Processes*

Volume 8   *Private Fostering and Miscellaneous*

Volume 9   *Adoption Issues*

These give authoritative guidance about the intentions and requirements of the Children Act 1989 and generate a comprehensive picture of its impact on professional practice.

171 A series of texts on the Children Act have been published. For example, A Guide to The Children Act 1989 (White, Carr and Lowe) was published in 1990. This is now in an expanded and updated second edition, The Children Act in Practice (White, Carr and Lowe, 1995). Each edition contains a commentary on the main provisions. The second edition reproduces the Act, as amended, in full. Various training packs have been produced by statutory, voluntary and educational bodies. These include the Open University, the National Children's Bureau, and the Department of Health.

172 Additionally, the NHS Health Advisory Service has published a number of texts that are of direct relevance to commissioning, purchasing and providing mental health services for children and adolescents. These are:

- *Suicide Prevention - The Challenge Confronted*, ISBN 011 321821 4, 1994. London: HMSO.

- *Together We Stand - The Commissioning Role and Management of Child and Adolescent Mental Health Services*, ISBN 011 321904 0, 1995. London: HMSO.

- *A Place in Mind - Commissioning and Providing Mental Health Services for People Who Are Homeless*, ISBN 011 321925 3, 1995. London: HMSO.

- *The Substance of Young Needs - Commissioning and Providing Services for Children and Adolescents Who Use and Misuse Substances*, ISBN 0 11 321934 2, 1996. London: HMSO.

173 Each of these books reports on the current challenges facing services and on their current capacities and capabilities. Each advises on good practice in commissioning and providing services and recommends ways in which that good practice can be implemented. Also, the constraints, challenges and enabling powers and duties, as framed by the law, are considered as are appropriate ways of putting good practice into effect within a lawful framework.

BIBLIOGRAPHY

Adcock M, White R, Hollows A, (eds.), 1991. *Significant Harm*. Croydon: Significant Publications.

Black D, Wolkind S, Harris Hendriks J, (eds.), 1991. *Child Psychiatry and the Law* (2nd edn.). London: Gaskell (Third edition expected 1996.)

British Medical Association and The Law Society, 1995. *Assessment of Mental Capacity - Guidance for Doctors and Lawyers.* London: BMA.

Department of Health, 1990. *The Care Programme Approach.* HC(90)28/LASSL(90)11.

Department of Health, 1991. *Welfare of Children and Young People in Hospital.* London: HMSO.

Department of Health, 1991. *The Care of Children - Principles and Practice in Regulations and Guidance.* London: HMSO.

Department of Health, 1991. *The Children Act 1989 - An Introductory Guide for the NHS.* London: HMSO.

Department of Health, 1991. *Patterns and Outcomes in Child Placement: Messages from Research and their Implications.* London: HMSO.

Department of Health, 1993. *Guidance on Permissible Forms of Control in Residential Care.*

Department of Health, 1995. *Child Protection - The Challenge of Partnership in Child Protection: Practice Guide.* London: HMSO.

Department of Health, 1995. *Child Protection: Messages from Research.* London: HMSO.

Department of Health, 1995. *Child Protection: Clarification of Arrangements between the NHS and other Agencies.* London: HMSO.

Department of Health, 1995. *Child Protection: Medical Responsibilities.* London: HMSO.

Department of Health and Welsh Office, 1990. *Code of Practice, Mental Health Act 1983.* London: HMSO.

Eekelaar J, Dingwall R, 1990. *The Reform of Child Care Law. A Practical Guide to the Children Act 1989*. London: Routledge.

Elton A, Hang P, Bentovim A, Simons J, 1995. *Withholding Consent to Life Saving Treatments: Three Cases*. British Medical Journal, 310.

Family Courts Consortium, 1991. *Information Pack and Bulletin*. London: FCC.

Harris Hendriks J, Richardson G, Williams R, 1990. *Ethical and Legal Issues*. In: *Child and Adolescent Psychiatry: Into the 1990s (OP 8)* (eds. D Black & J Harris Hendriks). London: Royal College of Psychiatrists.

Harris Hendriks J, Williams R, 1992. *The Children Act 1989 - England and Wales*. Journal of Child Psychology and Psychiatry. Review and Newsletter, 14,5, 213-220.

Hendrick J, 1993. *Child Care Law for Health Professionals*. Oxford: Radcliffe Medical Press.

Home Office, Department of Health, Department of Education and Science & Welsh Office, 1991. *Working Together Under the Children Act 1989. A Guide to Arrangements for Inter-agency Co-operation for the Protection of Children from Abuse*. London: HMSO.

Jones D, 1991. *Working with the Children Act: Tasks and Responsibilities of the Child and Adolescent Psychiatrist*. In: *Proceedings of the Children Act 1989 Course (OP12)* (ed. C Lindsey). London: Royal College of Psychiatrists.

Lord Chancellor's Department, 1991. *Family Proceedings Rules 1991*. London: HMSO.

Lord Chancellor's Department, 1991. *Family Proceedings Courts (Children Act 1989) Rules 1991*. London: HMSO.

Lord Chancellor's Department, 1991. *Children (Allocation of Proceedings) Order 1991*. London: HMSO.

Lord Chancellor's Department, *The Children Act Advisory Committee Reports, 1991-92, 1992-93, 1993-94, 1994-95 and 1995-96*.

National Children's Bureau, 1989. *The Children Act 1989. Highlight No. 91*. London: NCB.

National Children's Bureau, 1990. *Working with the Children Act 1989*. London: NCB.

NHS Management Executive, 1990. *Guidance on Consent to Examination and Treatment*. London: Department of Health.

Open University, 1991. *The Children Act 1989 - Putting it into Practice*. Milton Keynes: Open University.

Plotnikoff J, Woolfson R for Department of Health, 1996. *Reporting to Court under the Children Act*. London: HMSO.

Ruegger M, 1994. *Children's Rights in Relation to Giving and Withholding Treatment*. In: *Children and the Law.*, pp 43-49, (ed D L Lockton). De Montfort University Law School.

Spencer J R, Flin R, 1990. *The Evidence of Children*. London: Blackstone.

White R, Carr P, Lowe N, 1995. *The Children Act 1989 in Practice*. London: Butterworths.

Williams R, Harris Hendriks J, 1991. *Introducing the Children Act 1989*. General Practitioner, 18 October 1991, 52-58.

Williams R, Harris Hendriks J, 1992. *Introducing the Children Act 1989*. In: *The Law and General Practice* (ed. D. Pickersgill). Oxford: Radcliffe Medical Press.

*An Index of Orders
and Sections*

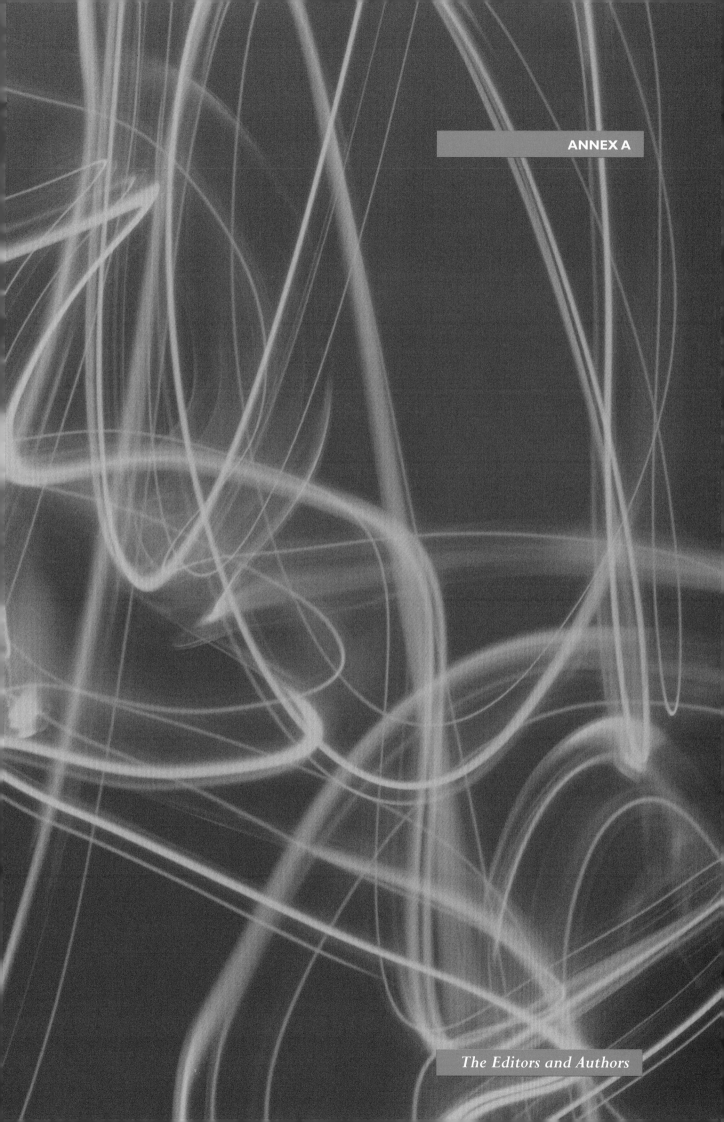

The Editors and Authors

Mr Richard White

Richard White was admitted as a solicitor in 1972. He has worked in a local authority and as a research director at the British Agencies for Adoption and Fostering. Since 1986, he as been a partner in White and Sherwin, solicitors of Croydon. The practice specialises in the law relating to children. He is co-author of the *Children Act in Practice*, (1995), and the *Concise Guide to the Children Act (1989)*, and editor of *Clarke Hall and Morrison*, an encyclopaedia on child law. He was a member of the NHS Health Advisory Service/Mental Health Act Commission/Social Services Inspectorate Team which reviewed adolescent forensic mental health services in 1993-94.

Dr Richard Williams

Richard Williams is the present Director of the NHS Health Advisory Service (HAS). Upon appointment in 1992, he was required to reposition the HAS so that it could exercise its remit within the reformed health service. He has developed four new roles for the HAS.

Since 1980, he has been a consultant child and adolescent psychiatrist at the Bristol Royal Hospital for Sick Children, where he developed an extensive liaison and consultation practice with other community child care workers and the child health services. His particular clinical interests include the psychological impacts and psychiatric treatment of life-threatening and chronic physical disorders and the immediate and long-term management of psychological trauma in families.

Outside his clinical role and throughout the past 14 years, he has developed specialised experience in selecting and training leaders. Richard Williams has been involved in service management and, consequent on his work with the HAS, has gained particular experience with the challenges posed to health and local authorities and general practitioners in commissioning comprehensive health services for mentally ill and elderly people.

Mr William Bingley

William Bingley is a lawyer by training. From 1983 to 1989, he was Legal Director of MIND (National Association for Mental Health). In 1989, he was seconded to the Department of Health to act as Executive Secretary of the Working Group which prepared the Mental Health Act Code of Practice, published in 1990. In the same year, he became the first Chief Executive of the Mental Health Act Commission, a post which he still holds.

William Bingley is a co-opted member of the BMA Medical Ethics Committee and has observer status on the Law Society's Mental Health and Disability Sub-Committee. In 1992, he was appointed a member of the Department of Health Working Group on The Future of High Security and Related Psychiatric Provision.

Mr Anthony Harbour

Anthony Harbour was admitted as a solicitor in 1980. He is a member of two Law Society specialist panels -the Mental Health and Children Panels. He has worked both in private practice and for local authorities. He has extensive experience in children's law - representing local authorities, parents and children. He also has substantial experience of representing mentally ill people. He has advised local authorities and health authorities concerning mental health and child care matters. He has a particular interest in the problems of children involved with the mental health services. He regularly trains social workers and health care professionals on child and mental health law topics. He also writes on many aspects of the law relating to children and mental health.

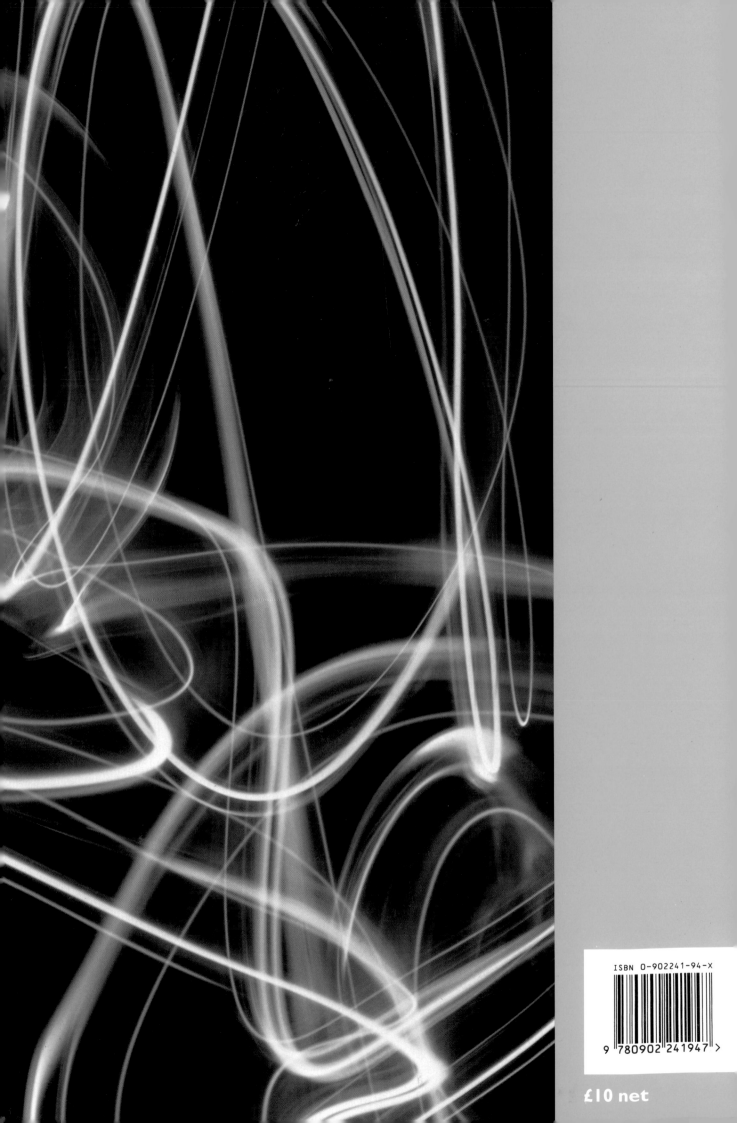

ISBN 0-902241-94-X

9 780902 241947 >

£10 net

TRUE TO LIFE

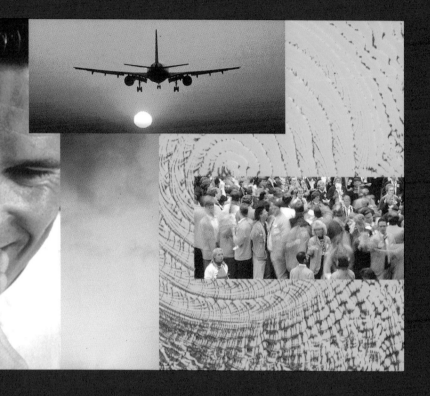

PRE-INTERMEDIATE

Ruth Gairns
Stuart Redman

CLASS BOOK

CAMBRIDGE
UNIVERSITY PRESS